Lecture Notes of the Institute
for Computer Sciences, Social Informatics
and Telecommunications Engineering 639

Editorial Board Members

Ozgur Akan, *Middle East Technical University, Ankara, Türkiye*
Paolo Bellavista, *University of Bologna, Bologna, Italy*
Jiannong Cao, *Hong Kong Polytechnic University, Hong Kong, Hong Kong*
Geoffrey Coulson, *Lancaster University, Lancaster, UK*
Falko Dressler, *University of Erlangen, Erlangen, Germany*
Domenico Ferrari, *Università Cattolica Piacenza, Piacenza, Italy*
Mario Gerla, *UCLA, Los Angeles, USA*
Hisashi Kobayashi, *Princeton University, Princeton, USA*
Sergio Palazzo, *University of Catania, Catania, Italy*
Sartaj Sahni, *University of Florida, Gainesville, USA*
Xuemin Shen, *University of Waterloo, Waterloo, Canada*
Mircea Stan, *University of Virginia, Charlottesville, USA*
Xiaohua Jia, *City University of Hong Kong, Kowloon, Hong Kong*
Albert Y. Zomaya, *University of Sydney, Sydney, Australia*

The LNICST series publishes ICST's conferences, symposia and workshops.
   LNICST reports state-of-the-art results in areas related to the scope of the Institute.
   The type of material published includes

- Proceedings (published in time for the respective event)
- Other edited monographs (such as project reports or invited volumes)

   LNICST topics span the following areas:

- General Computer Science
- E-Economy
- E-Medicine
- Knowledge Management
- Multimedia
- Operations, Management and Policy
- Social Informatics
- Systems

Utku Kose · Jafar Alzubi
Editors

IoT Technologies and Wearables for HealthCare

5th EAI International Conference, HealthWear 2024
Virtual Event, December 2–3, 2024
Proceedings

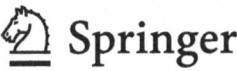

Editors
Utku Kose
Suleyman Demirel University
Isparta, Türkiye

Jafar Alzubi
Al-Balqa Applied University
Al-Salt, Jordan

ISSN 1867-8211 ISSN 1867-822X (electronic)
Lecture Notes of the Institute for Computer Sciences, Social Informatics
and Telecommunications Engineering
ISBN 978-3-031-95570-9 ISBN 978-3-031-95571-6 (eBook)
https://doi.org/10.1007/978-3-031-95571-6

© ICST Institute for Computer Sciences, Social Informatics and Telecommunications Engineering 2025

This work is subject to copyright. All rights are solely and exclusively licensed by the Publisher, whether the whole or part of the material is concerned, specifically the rights of translation, reprinting, reuse of illustrations, recitation, broadcasting, reproduction on microfilms or in any other physical way, and transmission or information storage and retrieval, electronic adaptation, computer software, or by similar or dissimilar methodology now known or hereafter developed.
The use of general descriptive names, registered names, trademarks, service marks, etc. in this publication does not imply, even in the absence of a specific statement, that such names are exempt from the relevant protective laws and regulations and therefore free for general use.
The publisher, the authors and the editors are safe to assume that the advice and information in this book are believed to be true and accurate at the date of publication. Neither the publisher nor the authors or the editors give a warranty, expressed or implied, with respect to the material contained herein or for any errors or omissions that may have been made. The publisher remains neutral with regard to jurisdictional claims in published maps and institutional affiliations.

This Springer imprint is published by the registered company Springer Nature Switzerland AG
The registered company address is: Gewerbestrasse 11, 6330 Cham, Switzerland

If disposing of this product, please recycle the paper.

Preface

It is a pleasure for us to introduce the proceedings of the fifth European Alliance for Innovation (EAI) International Conference on Wearables in Healthcare (HealthWear), held on December 2–3, 2024. The conference was held online and organized by Suleyman Demirel University, Turkey. EAI HealthWear highlights the pivotal role of wearable technologies in transforming healthcare and the fifth edition of the event considered the latest advancements in IoT, sensors, network infrastructure, intelligent algorithms and the associated communication mechanisms to ensure effective services/solutions for healthcare, through smart wearable systems. With a focus on cybersecurity, data privacy and usability, EAI HealthWear 2024 aimed to foster discussions on the secure, ethical and responsible use of wearables. The event brought together researchers, developers, experts and practitioners to discuss the latest advancements and future perspectives in terms of healthcare wearables.

The technical program of HealthWear included 12 full papers, accepted from 39 submissions after a double-blind review process in which submissions received three reviews each, and presented in oral presentation sessions. The proceedings cover all papers under three sections: Emerging Applications, Analysis Applications, and Cybersecurity. In addition to the high-quality technical paper presentations, the program also featured two keynote speeches. The two keynote speeches were given by Jose Antonio Marmolejo from National Autonomous University of Mexico, Mexico and Paniel Reyes Cárdenas from Oblate School of Theology, USA. Marmolejo presented a speech on development challenges regarding Digital Twins in healthcare while Cárdenas discussed care in the age of healthwear by rethinking responsibility and connection.

Coordination with the steering chairs, Nicola Francesco Lopomo and Paolo Perego, was critical for the success of HealthWear 2024. We sincerely appreciate their great support to make the event a total success. We are also grateful for the efforts of the valuable organizing committee team members. Also, we would like to thank the technical program committee members for their support in completing an objective peer-review processes of technical papers and providing a high-quality technical program. We would like to also thank Veronika Kissova from EAI for her endless support and guidance in organizing and coordinating the conference. Also, we are grateful to all authors for their valuable research works and presentations.

We are sure that the readers will find each paper in these proceedings a valuable and cutting-edge piece for understanding the present state of wearables and their place in healthcare applications. As also papers in these proceedings point out, wearables and the associated components have critical potential for advancing the future of healthcare. We are wide open to any ideas and feedback to advance future editions of EAI HealthWear.

Utku Kose
Jafar Alzubi

Organization

Steering Committee

Nicola Francesco Lopomo Politecnico di Milano, Italy
Paolo Perego Politecnico di Milano, Italy

Organizing Committee

General Chair

Utku Kose Süleyman Demirel University, Turkey

General Co-chair

Jose Antonio Marmolejo-Saucedo National Autonomous University of Mexico, Mexico

TPC Chairs

Utku Kose Süleyman Demirel University, Turkey
Jafar Alzubi Al-Balqa' Applied University, Jordan
Hakan Yuksel Isparta Applied Sciences University, Turkey

TPC Co-chair

Roman Rodriguez-Aguilar Universidad Panamericana, Mexico

Sponsorship and Exhibit Chair

Cem Deniz Kumral Isparta Applied Sciences University, Turkey

Local Chairs

Gül Fatma Türker	Süleyman Demirel University, Turkey
Gamze Köse	Aydin Adnan Menderes University, Turkey
Hakan Yüksel	Isparta Applied Sciences University, Turkey

Workshops Chair

Deepak Gupta — Maharaja Agrasen Institute of Technology, India

Publicity and Social Media Chair

Ibrahim Arda Cankaya — Süleyman Demirel University, Turkey

Web Chair

Dmytro Zubov — University of Central Asia, Kyrgyzstan

Technical Program Committee

Ashish Khanna	Maharaja Agrasen Institute of Technology, India
Bekir Aksoy	Isparta Applied Sciences University, Turkey
Bogdan Pătruţ	"Alexandru Ioan Cuza" University of Iaşi, Romania
Dmytro Zubov	University of Central Asia, Kyrgyzstan
Ecir Ugur Kucuksille	Süleyman Demirel University, Turkey
Hakan Yüksel	Isparta Applied Sciences University, Turkey
Junzo Watada	Waseda University, Japan
Rubaiyat Hossain Mondal	Bangladesh University of Engineering and Technology, Bangladesh
Mohamed Lahby	Hassan II University of Casablanca, Morocco
Neena Goveas	BITS Pilani, Goa Campus, India
Nga Nguyen	University of Wyoming, USA
Oluwasefunmi Arogundade	Federal University of Agriculture, Nigeria
Prakash Ranganathan	University of North Dakota, USA
Subrato Bharati	Concordia University, Canada
Uğur Güvenç	Düzce University, Turkey
Valentina E. Balas	Aurel Vlaicu University of Arad, Romania
Xi Chen	Meta, USA
Zongjie Wang	University of Connecticut, USA

Contents

Emerging Applications

Enhancing Remote Monitoring and Diagnosis of Heart Diseases Through IoT and Machine Learning Integration 3
   Shrawan Kumar and Bharti Thakur

CigEst: A Machine Learning-Based Wearable Device for Monitoring Smoking Habit 22
   Harish Kumar Rachuri, Ishna Jain, Rahul Dass, and Bharghava Rajaram

Digital Innovation for Individual Approach to Incorrect Spine Posture in Adolescents "NOVA-SPINE" 34
   Gabriele Pontillo, Claudio Catalano, Viviana Andreozzi, Luca Maresca, and Sara Liguori

Artificial Intelligence-Enabled Smart Glasses and Mobile Application for the Visually Impaired: Innovative Solutions in Wearable Health Technologies 47
   Bekir Aksoy, Mustafa Melikşah Özmen, and Muzaffer Eylence

Examining Personalized Explainable Recommendations that Support College Students on Stress Management 59
   Mamatha Putta and Jomara Sandbulte

Analysis Applications

Leveraging mHealth and Artificial Intelligence for Enhanced Health Indicators, A TwiMV Framework Proposal 87
   Domínguez-Miranda Sergio Arturo and Rodriguez-Aguilar Roman

Hardware Analysis for Low-Cost Wearable ECG Monitoring and Analysis System 108
   Shashank Rana, Aditya Handur-Kulkarni, Akhil Binu, Shubhangi Gawali, and Neena Goveas

A Method for Detecting Key Fiducial Points in Electrocardiographic Signals for Wave Characterization and HRV Analysis 117
   Luna Panni, Gloria Cosoli, and Lorenzo Scalise

A Minimum Routing Cost Algorithm Based on Quality of Service
in Wireless Mesh Networks 132
  Shufan Lin and Zsehong Tsai

Cybersecurity

Navigating Cybersecurity Challenges in Healthcare: Challenges,
Innovations, and EU Legal Framework for Connected Medical Devices 159
  Dusko Milojevic and Maja Nisevic

A Study and Assessment of the Importance of Cybersecurity in the Internet
of Things for Healthcare Wearables 182
  Mohammed Ridha Faisa Faisal

Integrating Artificial Intelligence and Cybersecurity in Healthcare
for the Advancements of Industry 5.0 198
  *Firoz Khan, Lakshmana Kumar Ramasamy, Emad Abd Al Rahman,
  and Amala Jayanthi*

Author Index 211

Emerging Applications

Enhancing Remote Monitoring and Diagnosis of Heart Diseases Through IoT and Machine Learning Integration

Shrawan Kumar and Bharti Thakur(✉)

Yogananda School of AI, Computer and Data Sciences, Shoolini University, Solan, H.P, India
bhartithakur.thakur@gmail.com

Abstract. Healthcare is undergoing a transformation thanks to the combination of Internet of Things (IoT) and machine learning (ML) technologies, particularly in the monitoring and detection of heart problems. The results of recent studies that use IoT and ML to improve cardiac health monitoring and predictive diagnoses are summarized in this review paper. The combination of machine learning (ML) with the Internet of Things (IoT) provides a promising path towards personalized treatment, early disease identification, and better cardiac disease management. Through a thorough assessment of the literature, including research that make use of wearable sensors, cloud-based data analytics, and deep learning algorithms, this paper illustrates the potential of IoT and ML to revolutionize cardiac healthcare. The advantages of remote monitoring systems—which offer ongoing health data, facilitating pre-emptive actions and lessening the need for in-person visits—are covered. This paper also discusses security concerns, data privacy, and the incorporation of these technologies into current healthcare systems. This paper highlights the usefulness of IoT and ML in detecting heart disease, improving patient outcomes, and opening the door for a more effective, economical healthcare system by looking at case studies and recent research findings. Future research directions are discussed in the paper's conclusion, with a focus on the necessity of scalable, secure, and patient-centred solutions in the continuing development of technology for heart disease monitoring and diagnostics.

Keywords: IoT (Internet of Things) · Machine Learning · Heart Disease Monitoring · Remote Healthcare · Wearable Technology · Data Privacy · Real-time Data Processing · Health Diagnostics · Cardiovascular Health · Predictive Analytics

1 Introduction

The convergence of Internet of Things (IoT) and machine learning (ML) technology is bringing about substantial improvements in more clinical and tailored interventions, especially in the monitoring and diagnosis of cardiovascular disorders. This change is driven by the urgent need to address the global problem of cardiovascular disease (CVD), which kills an estimated 17.9 million people a year and remains the leading cause of death worldwide [1, 2]. The traditional healthcare model, primarily reactive and based on periodic health check-ups and patient-reported symptoms, often results in delayed diagnosis and treatment of heart diseases. This delay can have fatal consequences, given the acute nature of many cardiac events. With the ability to continuously monitor and analyze patient health data in real-time, IoT and ML in healthcare promises to completely change this field and make it easier to identify and treat heart disease early [3]. A network of linked devices that can gather, share, and analyze data without the need for human interaction is referred to as the "Internet of Things" [4, 5]. IoT devices can be anything from implanted cardioverter-defibrillators to wearable heart rate monitors; all of these devices provide enormous volumes of real-time health data when it comes to monitoring heart disease. This data, when analyzed through ML algorithms, can provide unprecedented insights into a patient's health status, predict potential cardiac events, and enable personalized treatment plans [6, 7]. For instance, Predicts, an IoT and ML-based system, has demonstrated the capability to classify users into different risk levels of cardiovascular diseases (CVD) with significant accuracy, showcasing the potential of these technologies in enhancing cardiac care. Moreover, remote patient monitoring (RPM) systems (a group of IoT applications) have been shown to be effective in the management of cardiovascular disease, allowing doctors to monitor changes in blood pressure measurements and monitor patients' response to medications. This process not only improves patient outcomes but also reduces healthcare burden by reducing readmissions and increasing the ability for effective delivery [8]. Despite promising progress, integrating IoT and machine learning into cardiovascular care is not difficult. Significant hurdles include things like device integration, data privacy and security, and the requirement for reliable systems for data processing and storage [9–11]. Additionally, the accuracy and reliability of machine learning algorithms in cardiac diagnosis is still an area of ongoing research and development [12, 13] (Fig. 1).

This introduction sets the stage for a comprehensive exploration of how IoT and ML technologies are being applied to revolutionize the monitoring and diagnosis of heart diseases. It will delve into the current state of these technologies, their applications in cardiac care, the challenges faced in their implementation, and the future directions of this transformative integration. The final objective is to demonstrate how IoT and ML can be used to develop a more proactive, effective, and individualized healthcare system for individuals suffering from heart conditions.

Background

Heart Diseases: An Overview. Heart disease includes many diseases that affect the structure and function of the heart. Heart failure, arrhythmia, coronary artery disease, and issues with the heart valves are the main kinds. Symptoms range from no symptoms at all to life-threatening symptoms such as heart attack. The challenge is early detection and regular follow-up, as there are many heart diseases that have no early symptoms and therefore control is important to prevent major events [14, 15].

Internet of Things (IoT) in Healthcare. The usage of linked devices that gather and send health data in real-time is referred to as IoT in the healthcare industry. These devices range from wearable sensors to embedded medical devices, facilitating continuous patient

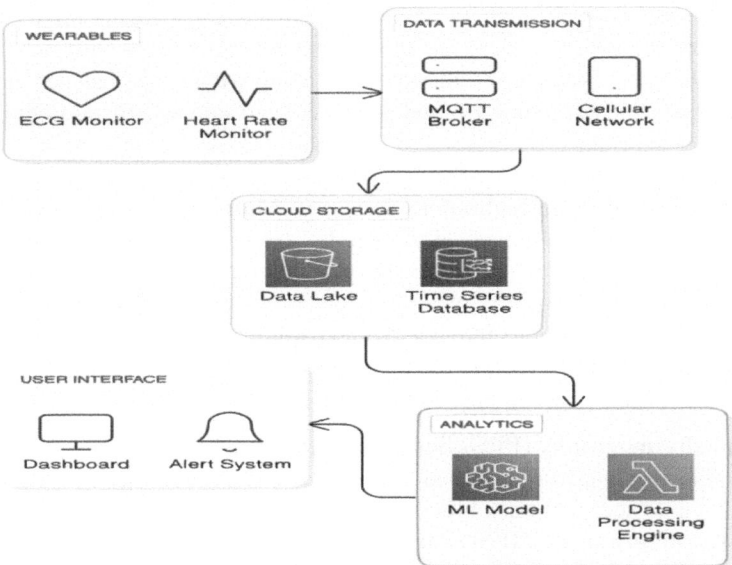

Fig. 1. Comprehensive flow of heart disease

monitoring outside traditional healthcare settings. Improved illness management through real-time data, increased patient engagement, and possibly cheaper healthcare costs by lowering the need for in-person visits and hospital stays are just a few benefits of the Internet of Things in the healthcare industry. Examples of IoT applications in heart disease monitoring include wearable ECG monitors and implantable devices that track heart rhythm and detect abnormalities early [16, 17].

Machine Learning in Healthcare. In the field of medicine, machine learning employs algorithms to evaluate enormous datasets in order to forecast results, identify diseases, and customize treatment regimens [18, 19]. Machine learning can improve diagnostic processes by identifying patterns in data that humans cannot see. Machine learning algorithms for heart disease analyze data from IoT devices to detect early signs of heart disease, predict patient outcomes, and improve treatment. Successful applications include algorithms that predict heart attacks from ECG data and systems that monitor heart failure patients to predict and prevent hospital readmissions [45, 46]. This background section sets the stage for a deeper exploration of how IoT and ML technologies are specifically applied to enhance the monitoring and diagnosis of heart diseases, addressing both the potential and the challenges of these innovative technologies.

2 IoT-Based Remote Monitoring for Heart Diseases

Wearable Devices and Sensors

One important application of IoT technology is the monitoring of cardiac problems through the use of wearables and sensors.

With their non-invasive and user-friendly design, these gadgets offer continuous health monitoring, which is especially important for individuals suffering from cardiovascular diseases. Wearable technology, including wristbands, patches, and smartwatches, has sensors that monitor blood pressure, heart rate, electrocardiogram (ECG) data, and other vital signs.
[20–22].

Overview of Wearable Technology for Heart Monitoring

Wearable technology has evolved to include devices capable of monitoring a wide range of physiological parameters. For instance, devices like the Fitbit Charge Heart Rate and the Oura Ring not only track physical activity but also monitor sleep patterns and heart rate, offering insights into the overall cardiovascular health of the user [22].

Types of Sensors Used in Wearable Devices

The sensors in wearable devices for heart disease monitoring typically include:

- **Photoplethysmography (PPG) Sensors:** They measure the variations in blood volume within the microvascular bed of tissue and are frequently found in wrist or finger-worn devices that track blood oxygen saturation and heart rate [9, 10].
- **Electrocardiogram (ECG) Sensors:** These are used to track the heart's electrical activity and are capable of identifying myocardial infarction, arrhythmias, and other cardiac disorders [10, 14].
- **Accelerometers:** Often used to monitor physical activity levels, these sensors can also help detect more subtle movements related to heart health and other physiological parameters [10].

Advantages and Limitations of Current Wearable Technologies

The primary advantage of wearable heart monitoring technologies is their ability to provide continuous, real-time data on a patient's cardiovascular health, which can be crucial for early detection of potential issues and management of chronic conditions. However, limitations exist, including issues with data accuracy, the need for frequent calibration, and user compliance in wearing the devices consistently [23, 24] (Fig. 2).

IoT Systems for Heart Health Monitoring

IoT systems for heart health monitoring involve not just the wearable devices themselves but also the infrastructure that supports the collection, transmission, and analysis of health data.

The Architecture of IoT-Based Systems

The typical architecture of an IoT-based heart health monitoring system includes wearable devices, a data transmission network, a cloud-based storage system, and an analytics platform that uses machine learning algorithms to interpret the data [25–27]. These systems are designed to be scalable and secure, ensuring that patient data is protected while providing valuable insights to healthcare providers.

Case Studies of IoT Systems in Action

Several case studies highlight the effectiveness of IoT systems in heart health monitoring:

- Remote Monitoring of Heart Failure Patients: Systems that monitor heart rate, blood pressure, and other vital signs have been shown to improve patient outcomes by allowing for timely interventions [12].

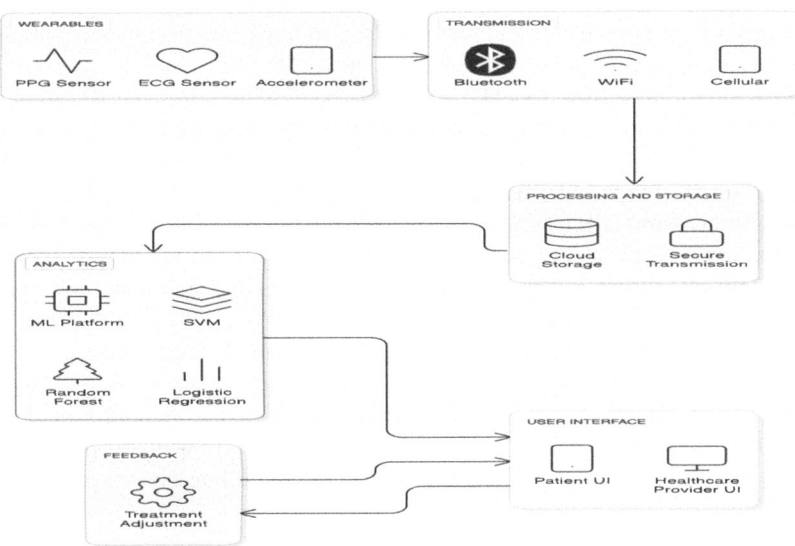

Fig. 2. T System for Heart Health Monitoring

- Detection and Management of Arrhythmias: IoT-based systems equipped with ECG sensors can detect abnormal heart rhythms and alert patients and doctors, facilitating early treatment [9, 11].

Challenges and Future Directions in IoT-Based Heart Health Monitoring

Although IoT-based systems have advantages, they face problems such as data privacy, the need for coordination between different devices and systems, and the ability to use technology. Future directions may include integrating more artificial intelligence algorithms to increase the predictive accuracy of these systems and developing more user-friendly tools to improve the patient's follow-up experience [9–12].

In Conclusion, IoT-based remote monitoring of heart diseases uses technology to provide valuable information regarding patients' cardiovascular health and enable good care, diagnosis and treatment of heart disease. But continued progress and solutions to current challenges are crucial to maximize the potential of this technology.

3 Machine Learning for Enhanced Diagnosis and Early Detection

By analysing large amounts of data to find patterns that human doctors are unable to see, machine learning (ML) algorithms facilitate earlier identification and better-informed diagnosis of cardiac disease. Among these methods are random forest (RF), logistic regression (LR), support vector machine (SVM), and others. Each algorithm has unique advantages in processing different data and diagnoses [9, 27–33].

Overview of Machine Learning Algorithms Used in Heart Disease Diagnosis

- **Random Forest (RF):** Because of its robustness against overfitting and capacity to handle huge datasets, RF has demonstrated improved performance in the prediction of

cardiac disease. Studies have demonstrated RF's effectiveness in enhancing predictive accuracy and reliability in heart disease diagnosis [28, 30].
- **Support Vector Machine (SVM):** SVM has been widely utilized to differentiate between healthy and ill cases based on heart disease signs since it is especially useful in classification jobs. It is valued for its high accuracy and the ability to model complex nonlinear relationships [27, 29, 31, 34].
- **Logistic Regression (LR):** When dealing with binary classification issues, like determining whether heart disease is present or not, LR is frequently utilized. It provides easily interpretable criteria, making it useful in clinical decision making [27].

Comparative Analysis of Machine Learning Algorithms Effectiveness

Research contrasting these algorithms' outputs has demonstrated that RF typically performs better than other algorithms in terms of accuracy and handling inconsistent data, including clinical data [28, 30]. SVM and LR also perform well, especially on data sets where the relationship between variables is clearly and linearly separated [27, 29, 31, 34].

Integration of Machine Learning with IoT Data

Integrating machine learning algorithms with data collected from IoT devices offers a promising way to improve diagnosis and early detection of heart disease. This integration allows for immediate data analysis and instant feedback, which is important in situations requiring urgent treatment.

Techniques for Combining IoT Data with Machine Learning Algorithms

Data Preprocessing: Before integration, data collected from IoT devices must be pre-processed to ensure quality and consistency. This includes cleaning, normalization, and transformation of data to fit the requirements of ML algorithms [30, 32, 33].

Feature Selection: Machine learning models can function better when the key properties from IoT data are chosen. Principal component analysis (PCA) and factor analysis of RF models are two often utilized techniques [30, 32, 33].

Challenges in Data Collection, Processing, and Analysis

Security and Privacy of Data: Ensuring the security and privacy of health data gathered by Internet of Things devices is a challenging task. To solve these problems, strong encryption and data anonymization technologies are required [30, 32, 33].

Data heterogeneity and data volume: IoT devices generate large amounts of data and different types, which require complex processes to process large volumes of data without impacting performance [30, 32, 33] (Fig. 3).

Examples of Successful Integrations and Their Outcomes

Heart Failure Prediction: Integrating ML with IoT has enabled predictive models that can forecast heart failure events by analysing real-time data from cardiac monitors. These models help in administering preventive measures proactively [30, 32, 33].

Arrhythmia Detection: Arrhythmias have been successfully detected by ML models combined with ECG data from wearable devices more quickly and correctly than with conventional techniques [30, 32, 33].

To sum up, machine learning holds promise for enhancing cardiac illness diagnostics and early detection. Using machine learning algorithms combined with IoT data, doctors

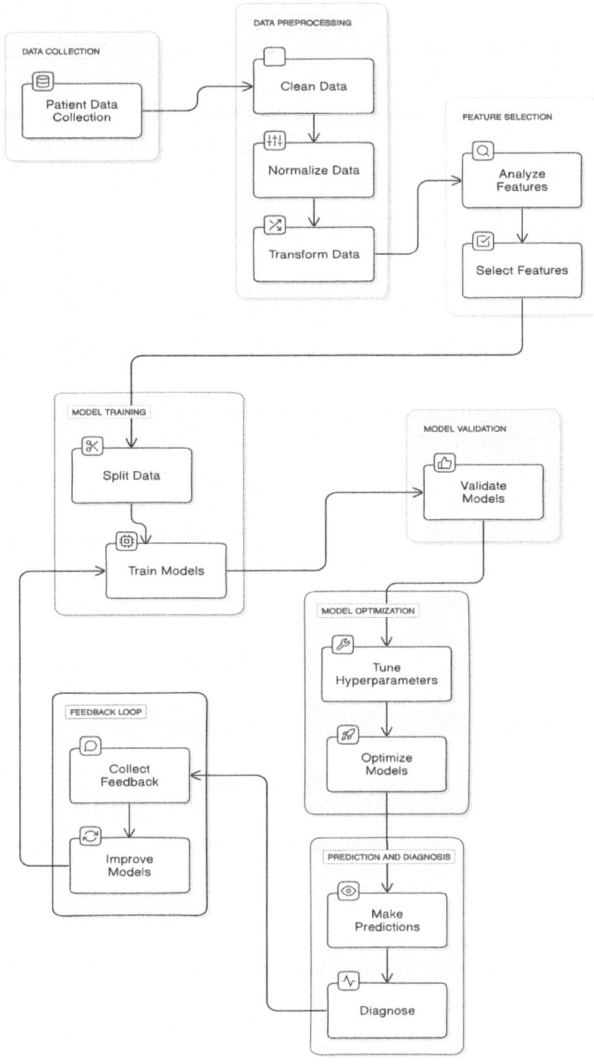

Fig. 3. Prediction cum Monitoring using IOT of Heart Disease

can achieve more accurate diagnosis, personalized treatment based on the patient's needs, and ultimately improve patient benefit. However, to realize the device's benefits, issues such as data privacy, performance, and integration with existing treatments need to be addressed.

Algorithms

The proposed work applied logistic regression, decision tree and support vector machine for the detection of heart disease from ECG signal. In this section, we will discuss all of these algorithms.

Logistic Regression

The logistic regression is the binary classifier which classifies the input features into two classes i.e. 0 and 1. The class 0 is the class where non-diseased features are classified as per the proposed work. In class 1, all the features of ECG come which contain some irregular patterns that point towards heart disease. It is probabilistic approach to classify the features in 0 and 1 classes. The equation of logistic equation is given below:

$$P(x) = \frac{1}{1 + e^{-(\beta_0 + \beta_1 x)}} \tag{1}$$

Here, in Eq. 1, P is the probability of belongingness of feature x in class 0 or 1. β_0 signifies the intercept and β_1 signifies the slope of the mode. The model forms 'S' curve from 0 to 1. The threshold value is 0.5 set to control the classification task.

Decision Tree

The decision trees classifier uses tree like structure to translate the training of features in the model. It discovers nodes based on information gain of the feature category. High information node contains high significant features for the dedicated task. Such nodes become root node or parent node. Leaves nodes or child nodes are those which contain low significant feature category for the dedication predictor values. The information gain (I.G) of each feature category is calculated as:

$$\text{I.G} = \text{Entropy} - \sum_{i=1}^{n} \left(\frac{D_i}{D} * Entropy(D_i)\right) \tag{2}$$

$$\text{Entropy} = -\sum_{i=1}^{n} p_i \log_2(p_i) \tag{3}$$

Equation 2 is used to measuring information gain in nodes containing feature category. Here, D_i is the subset dataset of D dataset. The entropy in Eq. 3 is used to measure the impurity in the dataset. Here, p_i is the probability of a feature classified in a particular class.

Support Vector Machine

Support vector machine has been used in the proposed work for the classification of ECG features into two classes i.e. diseased and non-diseased class. We have used linear kernel to draw linear hyperplane for making the linear discrimination among the features vectors of ECG data in X-Y plane. The linear kernel generates linear hyperplane that tries to fit best in X-Y place to separate the features of having irregularity and normal in ECG dataset. The linear hyperplane follow Eq. 4 given below.

$$w^T x + b = 0 \tag{4}$$

Here, w is normal vector to hyperplane. The b represents the offset value which is the distance of the hyperplane from the origin along the normal vector w. The SVM linear classifier model classifies the features in two classes considering as 1 and 0. So, SVM performs classification of ECG features in diseased class as 1 when $w^T x + b \geq 0$ otherwise the SVM classifies the features in non-diseased class as 0.

4 Machine Learning for Enhanced Diagnosis and Early Detection

The integration of cloud computing and big data analytics into heart disease monitoring and diagnosis represents a significant leap forward in healthcare technology. Cloud computing provides a scalable and efficient platform for storing and processing the vast amounts of data generated by IoT devices and healthcare systems. This is crucial for heart disease monitoring, where continuous data collection from wearable devices and remote monitoring systems generates large datasets that require substantial computational resources to analyse [23].

Big data analytics refers to advanced analytical techniques used to process and analyse this big data to obtain meaningful insights. Big data analytics can be used to find patterns, trends, and linkages in data that may point to the beginning or development of cardiac disease. For example, the health-Cloud system uses cloud computing and machine learning to accurately predict heart disease, enabling early intervention and behaviour change to prevent disease [35].

These technologies work together to enable real-time monitoring and analysis of heart health, giving medical professionals the most recent data to help them make decisions. Moreover, it supports the development of predictive models that can forecast potential heart disease events, enhancing preventive care measures [36].

Intelligent Automation Beyond Machine Learning

Deep learning (DL), neural networks (ANN), and support vector machines (SVM) are just a few of the numerous methods that make up artificial intelligence (AI), which is far more diverse than traditional machine learning. The detection and treatment of cardiovascular disorders (CVD), such as heart failure, atrial fibrillation, and heart discomfort from stroke, may be expedited by this technology [37, 38].

Specifically, deep learning has demonstrated efficacy in processing visual data, including electrocardiograms and echocardiograms; nevertheless, this has resulted in the inability to diagnose malignant arrhythmia results and vascular illnesses [39, 40]. ANN and SVM are effective in handling large data sets such as nonlinear relationships; ANN performs better in evaluating ECG data, and SVM performs well in disease classification [41].

However, these AI methods still face issues such as overfitting, underfitting, and misspecification, which can affect their accuracy and reliability [42]. Despite these obstacles, cardiac intelligence clearly plays a crucial role in bettering illness classification and subtyping, predicting cardiovascular outcomes, and enhancing the efficacy of diagnostic instruments [43, 44].

Cardiovascular healthcare has a bright future thanks to the integration of cloud computing, big data analytics, and cutting-edge AI approaches into heart disease monitoring and diagnostics. Improved patient outcomes, tailored treatment regimens, and more precise forecasts are made possible by these technologies. However, achieving the full potential of these cutting-edge technologies in healthcare will depend on resolving ethical and data protection issues, guaranteeing system interoperability, and overcoming technological obstacles [18, 19].

5 Experimental Results

The suggested work's outcomes are presented in this section. This section presents the findings from every machine learning model used to identify cardiac disease. A common dataset comprising ECG data from both healthy and sick individuals has been subjected to applications of logistic regression, decision trees, and support vector machines. Figure 4 shows the heat map of the feature vector which have been extracted from the ECG patterns.

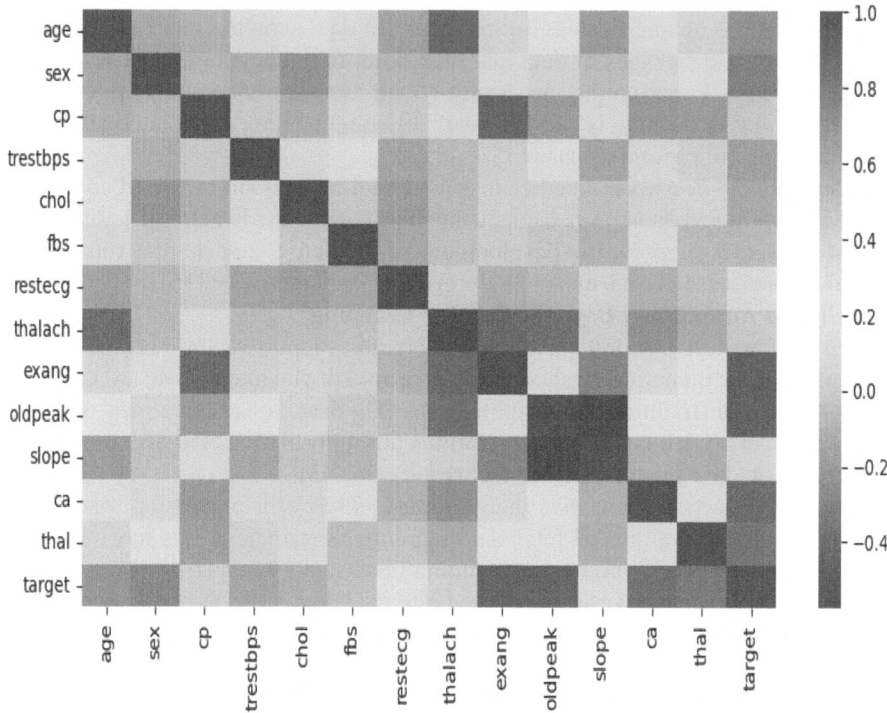

Fig. 4. Heap map of feature vector

Figure 4 shows the correlation among the feature vector of the ECG patterns. It helps to analyses the variation of energy components of the unique ECG patterns and helps to determine the irregular fluctuation in the heart signal. The frequency variation of the ECG signal in males and females according to age is depicted in Fig. 5.

Figure 5 helps us to determine the frequency change of ECG patterns in various age group among male and female population. Thiis helps to collect relevant data from the source and to mitigate irregularities in sampling process. The logistic regression model's performance is displayed in Fig. 6.

The logistic regression model has achieved an accuracy of 79.51%, recall of 87.38%, and F1 score of 81.08%, as illustrated in Fig. 5. The decision tree model's performance evaluation is displayed in Fig. 7.

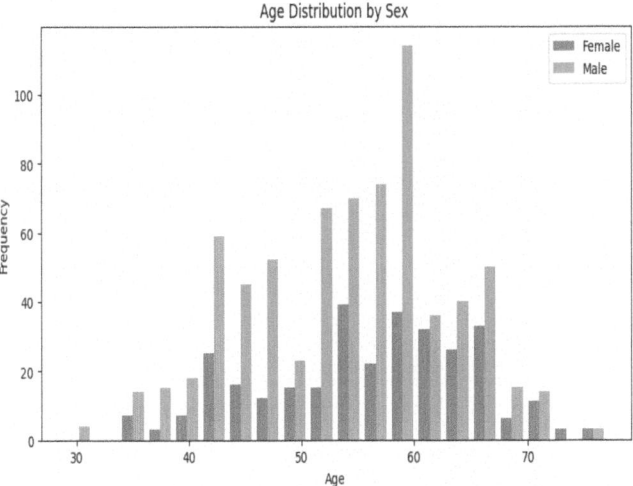

Fig. 5. Frequency change in ECG signal in male and female with respect to their age

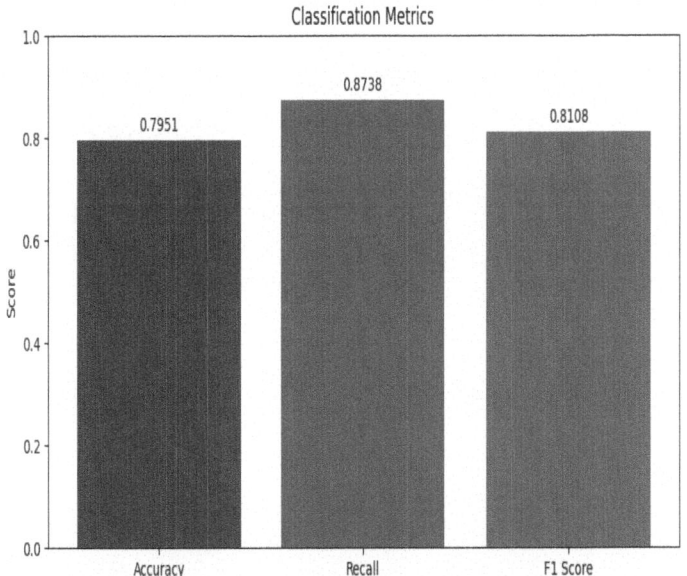

Fig. 6. Performance of logistic regression model

Figure 6 shows the accuracy of 98.54%, recall of 97.09% and F1 score of 98.52% have been attained by the decision tree model. The SVM model's performance evaluation is displayed in Fig. 8.

Figure 7 shows the accuracy of 88.78%, recall of 94.17% and F1 score of 89.4% have been attained by the SVM model. The ROC curve performance evaluation of each tree model is displayed in Fig. 9.

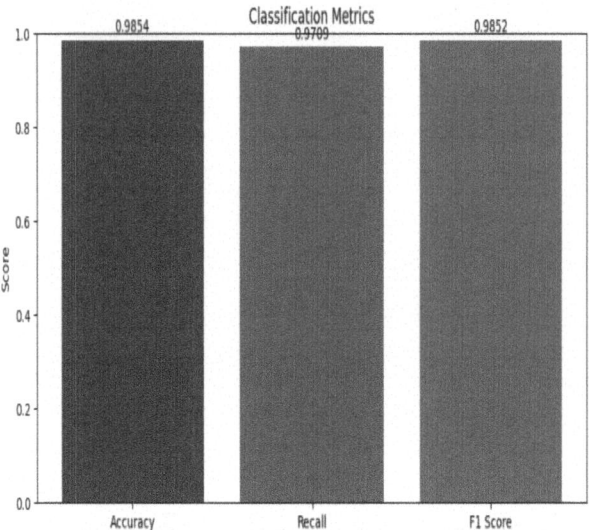

Fig. 7. Performance of decision tree model

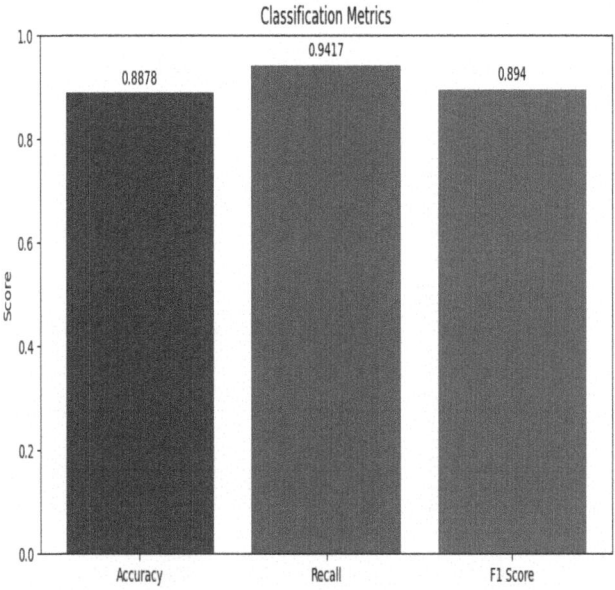

Fig. 8. Performance of SVM model

A comparison of the three models in terms of the ROC curve is presented in Fig. 8, which indicates that the decision tree model is detecting heart disease with a higher degree of accuracy than the other two models. The comparison of the three models' overall accuracy is displayed in Fig. 10.

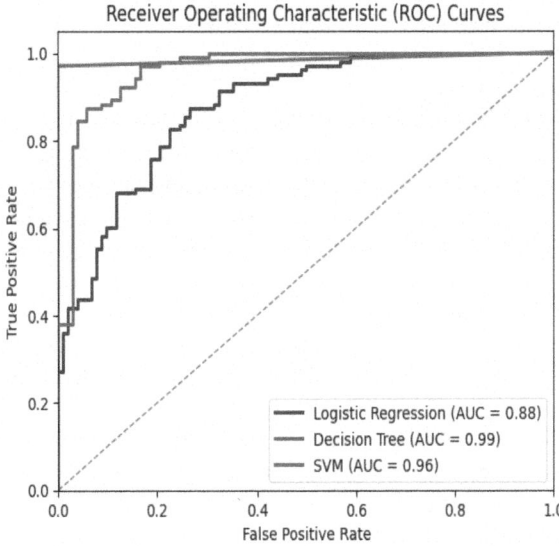

Fig. 9. The decision tree, logistic regression, and support vector machine models' ROC curves

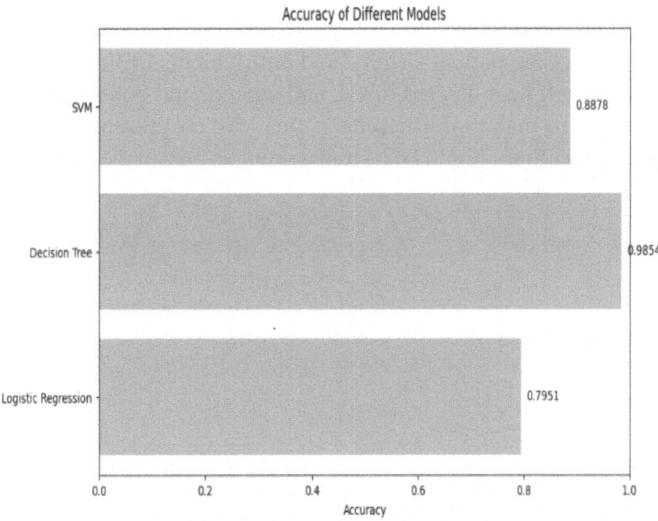

Fig. 10. Comparison of the accuracy of support vector machines, decision trees, and logistic regression

According to the Fig. 9 decision tress is generating higher accuracy of 98.54% for the detection of heart disease from ECG dataset. Consequently, the suggested study comes to the conclusion that the decision model performs better than the logistic regression and support vector machines.

6 Challenges and Ethical Considerations

Security and Privacy of Data

Data security and privacy are among the most crucial topics. The gathering, sending, and storing of health data via cloud and IoT technologies presents a serious danger of data leakage and inaccessibility [47–50]. The encryption and decryption process and other security measures are important but also present challenges and potential drawbacks [47]. Ensuring the privacy and security of patient information requires strong encryption methods, secure data transmission, and stringent controls [49, 50].

Reliability and Accuracy

Heart disease monitoring and prediction depend heavily on the dependability and precision of machine-learning techniques and connected devices. Inaccuracies in data collection or algorithmic predictions can lead to misdiagnoses or delayed treatment, potentially endangering patients' lives [48, 51, 52]. Ensuring the accuracy of machine learning predictions involves continuous validation against clinical outcomes and refining algorithms based on real-world performance [48, 51].

Algorithmic Bias and Fairness

Algorithmic bias is another important ethical issue. Machine learning models can unintentionally add bias to or augment data, leading to bias or discrimination [50].

Informed Consent and Transparency

Acceptance and transparency when using IoT and machine learning for cardiac care are important to respect the patient's rights and entitlements [50]. Patients must understand how their data will be collected, used, and shared, and consent must be obtained based on their ability to make informed decisions [50]. Additionally, the operation of machine learning algorithms should be as transparent as possible to doctors and patients

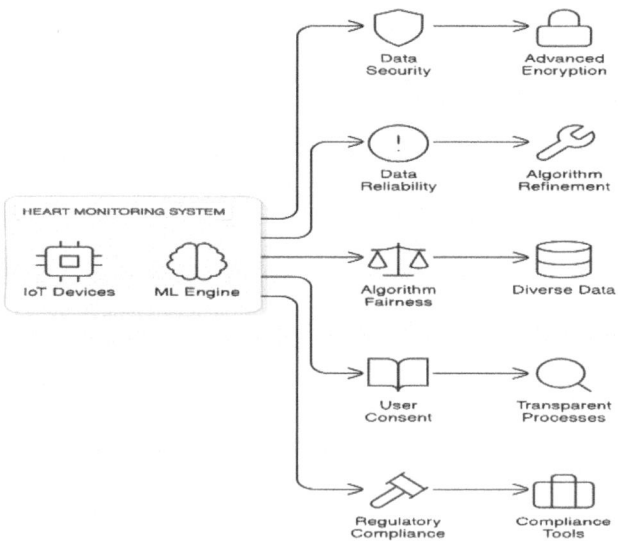

Fig. 11. Legal Challenges and Ethical Considerations

to ensure voluntary understanding and trust of decisions based on this technology [50]. Figure 11 discusses the Legal Challenges and Ethical Considerations.

Realizing technology's promise to enhance patient outcomes and healthcare requires ensuring data privacy and security, dependability and accuracy, integrity, consent, and legal compliance(Fig. 11).

7 Future Directions

Future directions in this field will focus on improving the capabilities of these technologies, addressing existing challenges, and exploring new applications to improve patient outcomes and healthcare efficiency.

Enhanced IoT Devices

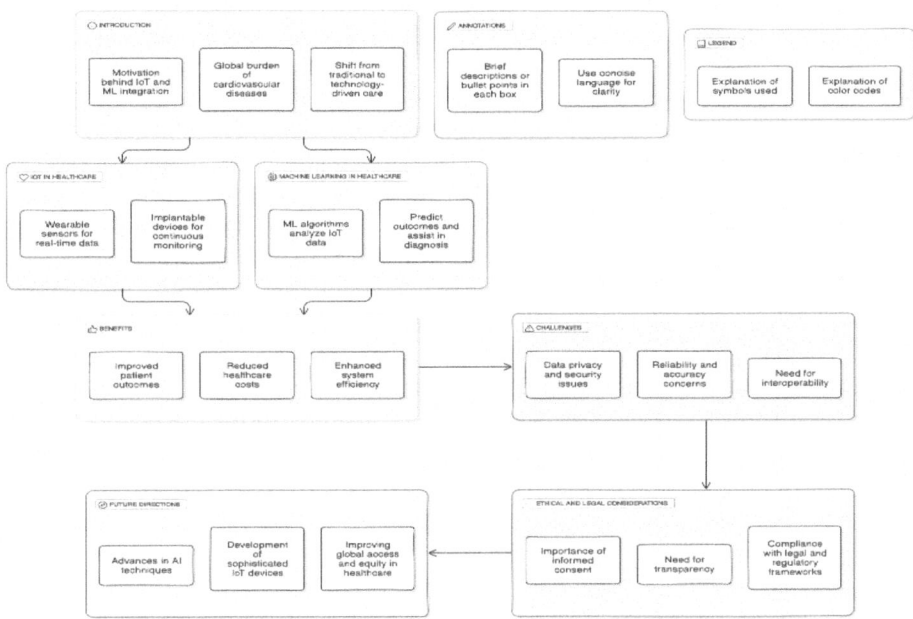

Fig. 12. The result of combining ML and IoT

IoT devices that can collect more health data should be developed. These tools will be designed to be more user-friendly, less invasive, and more efficient, leading to better understanding and better patient compliance [36, 37].

Integration Challenges and Solutions
Standardization and Interoperability

One of the key points of future development is the design of IoT devices and data entry to ensure interoperability of different systems and devices. This will facilitate the integration of IoT data with healthcare and facilitate the collection and analysis of data from different sources [38, 39].

Security Enhancements

Ensuring the security and privacy of the data that IoT devices store is still a major problem as these devices proliferate in the healthcare industry. Future studies should focus on the development of security systems and encryption systems to protect health information from cyber threats [40].

8 Conclusion

This paper explores the current state, benefits, challenges, and future directions of using IoT and machine learning to improve cardiovascular care and diagnosis. Thanks to detailed information and discussions of the latest scientific research, we see that this technology is evolving to revolutionize the treatment of heart diseases. From wearables to sensors, IoT devices can continuously track and monitor patients' heart health and provide valuable information for early detection and intervention impact.

However, realizing this potential is not without difficulties. Data privacy and security, device and algorithm reliability and accuracy, algorithm bias, and the need for collaboration between different systems are important issues that need to be addressed. Ethical considerations, including consent and transparency, as well as compliance with laws and regulations, also play an important role in fulfilling the responsibilities of IoT and machine learning in healthcare [54]. Additionally, solving ethical and regulatory issues, improving universal access and equity in healthcare, and reducing disparities in health outcomes clean drinking is an important goal to achieve [56].

The combination of IoT and machine learning holds great promise in revolutionizing cardiovascular care. By continuing to innovate and overcome challenges, we can unlock the full potential of these technologies to create clean healthcare that is more efficient, personalized and meaningful. The road ahead is tough and challenging, but the potential rewards for patients and doctors are significant. As we move forward, it is important to focus on patient care to ensure that the benefits of these technological advances are seen safely and that justice and equity are achieved (Fig. 12).

References

1. Bansal, A., et al.: Remote health monitoring system for detecting cardiac disorders. IET Syst. Biol. **9**(6), 309–314 (2015). https://doi.org/10.1049/iet-syb.2015.0012. PMID:26577166;PMCID:PMC8687161
2. Brites, I.S.G., da Silva, L.M., Barbosa, J.L.V., Rigo, S.J., Correia, S.D., Leithardt, V.R.Q.: Machine learning and IoT applied to cardiovascular diseases identification through heart sounds: a literature review. Informatics **8**(4), 73 (2021). https://doi.org/10.3390/informatics8040073
3. Cuevas-Chávez, A., et al.: A Systematic review of machine learning and IoT applied to the prediction and monitoring of cardiovascular diseases. Healthcare **11**(16), 2240 (2023). https://doi.org/10.3390/healthcare11162240
4. Umer, M., Sadiq, S., Karamti, H., Karamti, W., Majeed, R., Nappi, M.: IoT based smart monitoring of patients' with acute heart failure. Sensors (Basel) **22**(7), 2431 (2022). https://doi.org/10.3390/s22072431. PMID:35408045;PMCID:PMC9003513

5. Umer, M., et al.: Heart failure patients monitoring using IoT-based remote monitoring system. Sci. Rep. **13**(1), 19213 (2023). https://doi.org/10.1038/s41598-023-46322-6. PMID:37932424;PMCID:PMC10628138
6. Ziryawulawo, A., Ogare, A.C., Ayebare, F., Sinde, R.: Application of IoT and machine learning techniques for heart disease prediction and diagnosis: a comprehensive review. Int. J. Adv. Sci. Res. Eng. **08** (2022). https://doi.org/10.31695/IJASRE.2022.8.7.7
7. Fayoumi, A., BinSalman, K.: Effective remote monitoring system for heart disease patients (2018). https://doi.org/10.1109/CBI.2018.10056
8. Palumbo, A., Gramigna, V., Calabrese, B., Ielpo, N., Fragomeni, G.: A real-time remote monitoring system for cardiovascular diseases. Int. J. Eng. Trends Technol. **70**(11), 117–128 (2022). Crossref, https://doi.org/10.14445/22315381/IJETT-V70I11P212
9. Armand, T.P.T., Mozumder, M.A.I., Ali, S., Amaechi, A.O., Kim, H.C.: Developing a low-cost IoT-based remote cardiovascular patient monitoring system in Cameroon. Healthc. (Basel). **11**(2), 199 (2023). https://doi.org/10.3390/healthcare11020199. PMID:36673567;PMCID:PMC9859308
10. Prieto-Avalos, G., Cruz-Ramos, N.A., Alor-Hernández, G., Sánchez-Cervantes, J.L., Rodríguez-Mazahua, L., Guarneros-Nolasco, L.R.: Wearable devices for physical monitoring of heart: a review. Biosensors (Basel) **12**(5), 292 (2022). https://doi.org/10.3390/bios12050292. PMID:35624593;PMCID:PMC9138373
11. Almujally, N.A., et al.: Monitoring acute heart failure patients using internet-of-things-based smart monitoring system. Sensors (Basel) **23**(10), 4580 (2023). https://doi.org/10.3390/s23104580. PMID:37430494;PMCID:PMC10221603
12. Javeed, A., Zhou, S., Yongjian, L., Qasim, I., Noor, A., Nour, R.: An intelligent learning system based on random search algorithm and optimized random forest model for improved heart disease detection. IEEE Access **7**, 180235–180243 (2019)
13. Moshawrab, M., Adda, M., Bouzouane, A., Ibrahim, H., Raad, A.: Smart wearables for the detection of cardiovascular diseases: a systematic literature review. Sensors. **23**(2), 828 (2023). https://doi.org/10.3390/s23020828
14. Bayoumy, K., Gaber, M., Elshafeey, A., et al.: Smart wearable devices in cardiovascular care: where we are and how to move forward. Nat. Rev. Cardiol. **18**, 581–599 (2021). https://doi.org/10.1038/s41569-021-00522-7
15. Sun, X., Yin, Y., Yang, Q., et al.: Artificial intelligence in cardiovascular diseases: diagnostic and therapeutic perspectives. Eur. J. Med. Res. **28**, 242 (2023). https://doi.org/10.1186/s40001-023-01065-y
16. Karatzia, L., Aung, N., Aksentijevic, D.: Artificial intelligence in cardiology: hope for the future and power for the present. Front. Cardiovasc. Med. **9**, 645726 (2022). https://www.frontiersin.org/journals/cardiovascular-medicine/articles/10.3389/fcvm.2022.945726/full, https://doi.org/10.3389/fcvm.2022.945726, ISSN=2297-055X
17. Nancy, A.A., Ravindran, D., Raj Vincent, P.M.D., Srinivasan, K., Gutierrez, R.D.: IoT-cloud-based smart healthcare monitoring system for heart disease prediction via deep learning. Electronics **11**(15), 2292 (2022). https://doi.org/10.3390/electronics11152292
18. Yasmin, F., et al.: Artificial intelligence in the diagnosis and detection of heart failure: the past, present, and future. Rev. Cardiovasc. Med. **22**, 1095–1113 (2021). https://doi.org/10.31083/j.rcm2204121
19. Vaishali, G., Kalaivani, V.: Big data analysis for heart disease detection system using map reduce technique, pp. 1–6 (2016). https://doi.org/10.1109/ICCTIDE.2016.7725360
20. Nashif, S., Raihan, M., Islam, M., Imam, M.H.: Heart disease detection by using machine learning algorithms and a real-time cardiovascular health monitoring system. World J. Eng. Technol. **6**, 854–873 (2018). https://doi.org/10.4236/wjet.2018.64057
21. Yılmaz, R., Yağın, F.H.: Early detection of coronary heart disease based on machine learning methods. Med. Rec. **4**(1), 1–6 (2022)

22. Ketu, S., Mishra, P.K.: Empirical analysis of machine learning algorithms on imbalance electrocardiogram based arrhythmia dataset for heart disease detection. Arab. J. Sci. Eng. **47**(2), 1447–1469 (2022)
23. Patro, S.P., Padhy, N.: A secure IoT-cloud based remote health monitoring for heart disease prediction using machine learning and deep learning techniques. Eng. Proc. **56**(1), 241 (2023). https://doi.org/10.3390/ASEC2023-16580
24. Vandenberk, B., Chew, D.S., Prasana, D., Gupta, S., Exner, D.V.: Successes and challenges of artificial intelligence in cardiology. Front. Digit. Health. **28**(5), 1201392 (2023). https://doi.org/10.3389/fdgth.2023.1201392. PMID:37448836;PMCID:PMC10336354
25. Chang, V., Bhavani, V.R., Xu, A.Q., Hossain, M.A.: An artificial intelligence model for heart disease detection using machine learning algorithms. Healthc. Anal. **2**, 100016 (2022)
26. Chavda, P., Bhavsar, H., Pithadia, Y., Kotecha, R.: Early detection of cardiac disease using machine learning. In: 2nd International Conference on Advances in Science & Technology (ICAST) 2019 on 8th, 9th April 2019 by K J Somaiya Institute of Engineering & Information Technology, Mumbai, India (2019). SSRN: https://ssrn.com/abstract=3370813 or https://doi.org/10.2139/ssrn.3370813
27. Nagavelli, U., Samanta, D., Chakraborty, P.: Machine learning technology-based heart disease detection models. J. Healthc. Eng. **27**(2022), 7351061 (2022). https://doi.org/10.1155/2022/7351061. PMID:35265303;PMCID:PMC8898839
28. Bhatt, C.M., Patel, P., Ghetia, T., Mazzeo, P.L.: Effective heart disease prediction using machine learning techniques. Algorithms. **16**(2), 88 (2023). https://doi.org/10.3390/a16020088
29. Ahmad, A.A., Polat, H.: Prediction of heart disease based on machine learning using jellyfish optimization algorithm. Diagnostics (Basel). **13**(14), 2392 (2023). https://doi.org/10.3390/diagnostics13142392. PMID:37510136;PMCID:PMC10378171
30. Baghdadi, N.A., Farghaly Abdelaliem, S.M., Malki, A., et al.: Advanced machine learning techniques for cardiovascular disease early detection and diagnosis. J. Big Data **10**, 144 (2023). https://doi.org/10.1186/s40537-023-00817-1
31. Pandey, A., Shivaji, B.A., Acharya, M., Mohbey, K.K.: Mitigating class imbalance in heart disease detection with machine learning. Multimedia Tools Appl., 1–26 (2024)
32. Srinivasan, S., Gunasekaran, S., Mathivanan, S.K., et al.: An active learning machine technique based prediction of cardiovascular heart disease from UCI-repository database. Sci. Rep. **13**, 13588 (2023). https://doi.org/10.1038/s41598-023-40717-1
33. Uddin, K.M.M., Ripa, R., Yeasmin, N., Biswas, N., Dey, S.K.: Machine learning-based approach to the diagnosis of cardiovascular vascular disease using a combined dataset. Intell. Based Med. **7**, 100100 (2023). ISSN 2666-5212,https://doi.org/10.1016/j.ibmed.2023.100100
34. Mittelstadt, B.: Ethics of the health-related internet of things: a narrative review. Ethics Inf. Technol. **19**, 157–175 (2017). https://doi.org/10.1007/s10676-017-9426-4
35. Majhi, B., Kashyap, A.: Explainable AI-driven machine learning for heart disease detection using ECG signal. Appl. Soft Comput. **167**, 112225 (2024)
36. Gerke, S., Minssen, T., Cohen, G.: Ethical and legal challenges of artificial intelligence-driven healthcare. Artif. Intell. Healthc., 295–336 (2020). https://doi.org/10.1016/B978-0-12-818438-7.00012-5. Epub 2020 Jun 26. PMCID: PMC7332220
37. Kumar, M., et al.: Healthcare internet of things (H-IoT): current trends, future prospects, applications, challenges, and security issues. Electronics **12**(9), 2050 (2023). https://doi.org/10.3390/electronics12092050
38. Singh, A.K., Kumar, A., Kumar, V., Prakash, S.: COVID-19 Detection using adopted convolutional neural networks and high-performance computing. Multimedia Tools Appl. **83**(1), 593–608 (2024)

39. Das, R.C., Das, M.C., Hossain, M.A., Rahman, M.A., Hossen, M.H., Hasan, R.: Heart disease detection using ml. In: 2023 IEEE 13th Annual Computing and Communication Workshop and Conference (CCWC), pp. 0983–0987. IEEE (2023)
40. Ankit, K., Kumar, S.S., Navin, P.: A Deep Learning and powerful computational framework for brain cancer MRI image recognition. J. Inst. Eng. (India): Ser. B, **105**(1), 15–18 (2023)
41. Kumar, A., Chaurasia, B.K.: Detection of SARS-CoV-2 virus using lightweight convolutional neural networks. Wirel. Pers. Commun. **135**(2), 941–965 (2024)
42. Kumar, A., Singh, A.K., Singh, A., Kumar, V., Prakash, S., Tiwari, P.K.: An efficient framework for brain cancer identification using deep learning. Multimedia Tools Appl., 1–30 (2024). https://doi.org/10.1007/s11042-023-18017-7
43. Rajkumar, G., Gayathri Devi, T., Srinivasan, A.: Heart disease prediction using IoT based framework and improved deep learning. approach: medical application. Med. Eng. Phys. **111**, 103937 (2023). ISSN 1350-4533,https://doi.org/10.1016/j.medengphy.2022.103937
44. Davenport, T., Kalakota, R.: The potential for artificial intelligence in healthcare. Future Healthc. J. **6**(2), 94–98 (2019). https://doi.org/10.7861/futurehosp.6-2-94. PMID:31363513;PMCID:PMC6616181
45. Bohr, A., Memarzadeh, K.: The rise of artificial intelligence in healthcare applications. Artif. Intell. Healthc., 25–60 (2020). https://doi.org/10.1016/B978-0-12-818438-7.00002-2. Epub 2020 Jun 26. PMCID: PMC7325854
46. Kumar, A., Shaun, M.A., Chaurasia, B.K.: Identification of psychological stress from speech signal using deep learning algorithm. e-Prime-Adv. Electr. Eng. Electron. Energy **9**, 100707 (2024)
47. Kumar, A., Godse, S., Kolekar, S., Saini, D.K.J.B., Pandita, D., Tiwari, P.: Decoding stress with computer vision-based approach using audio signals for psychological event identification during COVID-19. J. Electr. Syst. **20**(2), 2716–2727 (2024)
48. Kumar, A., Singh, S.K., Bhardwaj, I., Singh, P.K., Khanna, A., Brahma, B.: Audio spectrogram analysis in IoT paradigm for the classification of psychological-emotional characteristics. Int. J. Inf. Technol., 1–11 (2024)
49. Jahin, M.A., Masud, M.A., Mridha, M.F., Aung, Z., Dey, N.: KACQ-DCNN: uncertainty-aware interpretable kolmogorov-arnold classical-quantum dual-channel neural network for heart disease detection. arXiv preprint arXiv:2410.07446 (2024)
50. He, Q., Maag, A., Elchouemi, A.: Heart disease monitoring and predicting by using machine learning based on IoT technology. In: 2020 5th International Conference on Innovative Technologies in Intelligent Systems and Industrial Applications (CITISIA), Sydney, Australia, pp. 1–10 (2020). https://doi.org/10.1109/CITISIA50690.2020.9371772
51. Ramkumar, G., Seetha, J., Priyadarshini, R., Gopila, M., Saranya, G.: IoT-based patient monitoring system for predicting heart disease using deep learning. Measurement **218**, 113235 (2023). ISSN 0263-2241, https://doi.org/10.1016/j.measurement.2023.113235
52. Thakur, B., Gupta, G., Kumar, N.: Hybrid genetic model with ANOVA for predicting breast neoplasm using METABRIC gene data. Mater. Today Proc. **56**, 1847–1852 (2016)
53. Thakur, B., Kumar, N., Gupta, G.: Machine learning techniques with ANOVA for the prediction of breast cancer. Int. J. Adv. Technol. Eng. Explor. **9**(87), 232 (2022)
54. Thakur, B., Kumar, N.: Prediction, detection and recurrence of breast cancer using machine learning based on image and gene datasets. In: Recent Innovations in Computing: Proceedings of ICRIC 2021, vol. 1, 263–273 (2022)

CigEst: A Machine Learning-Based Wearable Device for Monitoring Smoking Habit

Harish Kumar Rachuri[1], Ishna Jain[1], Rahul Dass[2], and Bharghava Rajaram[1](✉)

[1] Ecole Centrale School of Engineering, Mahindra University, Hyderabad, India
{harish20peee001,se20uecm109,bharghava.rajaram}@mahindrauniversity.edu.in
[2] School of Media, Mahindra University, Hyderabad, India
rahul.dass@mahindrauniversity.edu.in

Abstract. This paper proposes a wearable device, *CigEst*, to estimate the number of cigarettes the wearer has smoked and alerts the wearer using haptic feedback and a mobile phone application. The requirement for such a device is obvious in the backdrop of a staggering $1.134 trillion cigarette market, and increasing health and financial risks associated with smoking. The wearable device presented in this paper, *CigEst*, is a proof of concept built around a Bluetooth-enabled microcontroller integrated with a 6-axis accelerometer and a carbon monoxide gas sensor. The movement of the hand when the wearer smokes, while not unique, is a repetitive pattern of bringing the hand to the mouth. This movement can be detected using an accelerometer. A dataset was created by having multiple wearers wear the device while smoking. A machine learning model was built using this accelerometer data, and is deployed on the wearable device by reducing the model. The carbon monoxide sensor is used to trigger the machine learning model, since the detected hand movement is not unique to smoking. The number of hand movements to the mouth is recorded and the number of cigarettes smoked is estimated using this data. The same is sent through a mobile phone to an IoT server for long term storage and further analysis. The smoking action detection algorithm shows a maximum of 95.5% accuracy in detecting a smoking action, and 88% on deployment of the ML model on the wearable device.

Keywords: Smart Health · Wearable · Embedded AI · Machine Learning · Edge device

1 Introduction

Cigarette smoking is injurious to health - this aphorism is quite commonplace across the globe. However, this warning has repeatedly been ignored by cigarette smokers who continue to puff away a large number of cigarettes in a day [27].

Cigarette consumption has turned into a trillion dollar market, with cigarette being sold in markets and streets in almost all parts of the world [13]. So much so that the availability of cigarettes is far higher than compared to access to essential commodities households need regularly.

Cigarette smoke contains over 4,000 harmful compounds, with 69 known to be carcinogenic. Smoke arises from poorly ignited fuel that forms a mixture of minuscule particles in the air. Consequently, this form of pollution poses a risk to human health. [18]. Cigarette smoking causes cancer of the mouth and throat, esophagus, stomach, colon, rectum, liver, pancreas, voice box (larynx), lung, trachea, bronchus, kidney and renal pelvis, urinary bladder, and cervix, and causes acute myeloid leukemia, among other breathing ailments.

Apart from the health risks, smoking also places a financial burden, particularly on the lesser affluent classes of society. The impact of smoking on household food security has been studied extensively [6].

In this backdrop, it is imperative to address the issue of smoking. There have been approaches in literature and practice based on financial policy making [23, 24] and media awareness [11,12].

This paper presents an engineering device-based approach to address the issue of smoking. The last few years have witnessed an explosion of smart wearable devices, particularly for health monitoring purpose. Smart watches [26] and smart rings [4] have become more commonplace, with their applications extending beyond health monitoring. The consumer acceptability to wearable devices makes it a viable approach to monitoring smoking habit as well. The paper presents a proof of concept design, implementation and evaluation of *CigEst*, a wearable device which uses a carbon monoxide sensor and accelerometer to estimate the number of cigarettes smoked by the wearer and alert them accordingly. For this purpose, the wearable employs a machine learning model deployed on the edge i.e. on the wearable itself. *CigEst* achieved an accuracy of 95.5% accuracy, which proves its efficacy. Apart from the alert system for the wearer, the data is also stored on an IoT server for long term predictive analytics for smoking related ailments.

In addition to health monitoring, the data that is gathered in real-time would also lead towards financial empowerment as the wearer would be able to visualize the expenditure their smoking habit translates into, and the resulting financial burden.

The rest of the paper is organized as follows: Sect. 2 presents existing approaches in developing devices to detect and/or monitor cigarette smoking. The proposed wearable device - *CigEst* is discussed in Sect. 3, followed by the data collection and model training process in Sect. 4. The evaluation results for the device is presented in Sect. 5, followed by the conclusion in Sect. 6.

2 Related Work

There have been several devices proposed in literature that address the issue of smoking. These range from environmental sensing devices, image processing, and wearables. We present a selection of these proposals to show the current state of work in monitoring smoking habit.

2.1 Using Environmental Sensors and Other Non-wearable Methods

Some of the proposed devices [10,16,30] [20] use gas sensors to sense smoke in the environment and raise alerts, or wirelessly transmit the sensed data to nearby devices or the cloud for further processing. These devices can be utilized for creating smoke free areas but do not address individual smoking habits.

Other non-wearable approaches include computer vision techniques to detect smoking action. Wu et al. [28] proposed a image processing approach using Hidden Markov Models (HMM) to detect smoking events in videos. Belsare et al. [5] proposed a deep learning framework aimed at detecting smoke inhalation with exceptional precision and quantifying smoke exposure in real-world scenarios has been outlined. This method requires video capture of the individual who is smoking.

There have also been handheld devices [1,2,7] that measure the amount of Carbon Monoxide (CO) that is exhaled to estimate the extent of smoking. These are either deployed in a smoker's natural environment, or a voluntary action that has to be performed by an individual and cannot provide real-time monitoring of smoking without being geographically constrained.

2.2 Wearable Devices

With regard to the wearable devices proposed in literature, most devices make use of accelerometers and/or respiratory sensors.

Senyurek et al. [21] proposed a device to detect smoking events by monitoring the regularity of hand gestures using a one-axis accelerometer worn on the wrist of the dominant hand. While the simplicity of the device is advantageous, it suffers from poor accuracy (49%).

Cole et al. [8] explored the efficacy of accelerometer sensors in smartwatches to detect smoking gestures. Their findings demonstrated that accelerometer-based systems achieve an 85%–95% accuracy rate in recognizing smoking gestures amid similar actions when utilizing Artificial Neural Networks (ANNs). The advantage of this proposal is that it uses stock smart watches, and no additional devices or sensors. The drawback, however, is that it used limited data, demonstrated the concept on only one smart watch, and has issues with power usage due to the requirement of continuous monitoring with a high sampling rate. A similar study was also performed by Shoaib et al. [22].

Ali et al. [3] proposed a chest wearable device to measure the respiration of an individual to detect smoking action with an 86.7% accuracy. Similarly, Lopez et al. [14] proposed a non-intrusive wearable sensor system called the Personal Automatic Cigarette Tracker (PACT), which recorded distinctive hand-to-mouth gestures, applied a support vector machine for pattern recognition and alterations in breathing patterns associated with cigarette smoking, using both a hand wearable and a chest wearable. They reported 87% accuracy in detecting a smoking action. The drawback of these devices is that they required a chest wearable to detect respiration patterns, making it cumbersome to use it in everyday life.

Tang et al. [25] proposed a device where smoking events and puffs detection were performed by using four three-axis accelerometers, at the dominant wrist, dominant upper arm, non-dominant wrist, and ankle. They reported a maximum F1-score of 0.79.

In the study performed by Raiff et al. [19], four six-axes accelerometers were used on the dominant arm of an individual. A support vector machine model used to predict cigarette smoking based on these feature sets generated a false positive rate between 0.07 and 0.2 for different subjects.

[17] The author proposes a method RisQ, a mobile solution that leverages a wristband containing a 9-axis inertial measurement unit to capture changes in the orientation of a person's arm, and a machine learning pipeline that processes this data to accurately detect smoking gestures and sessions in real-time. Their model reached an F1-score of 0.85.

The main drawback of most of these proposals is that the accuracy of using only inertial sensors for tracking a smoking action is limited. Augmenting them with chest wearable for monitoring respiration increases the complexity of the device and reduces wearability. In this paper, we propose an alternate approach which uses inertial sensors along with a gas sensor to reduce the inaccuracies of the methods proposed in literature.

3 CigEst: The Proposed Wearable Device

As mentioned in the previous sections, most wearable devices make use of inertial data collected by accelerometers in detecting hand-to-mouth gestures to determine whether the wearer is smoking or not. The major drawback of using only inertial data is reduced accuracy, and selectivity as several other hand gestures can imitate the smoking action. Some of these devices are also augmented with chest wearable for respiration monitoring to correlate with the hand movement for increased accuracy.

In the above context, this paper proposes *CigEst*, a wearable device which uses inertial sensing along with a carbon monoxide sensor to increase the selectivity of detecting a smoking action.

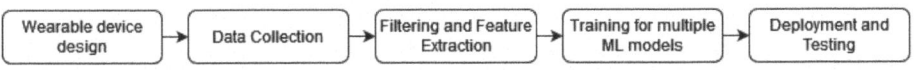

Fig. 1. Process flow for data collection, training, and testing

The design flow for the wearable is shown in Fig. 1. A hardware wearable device is built as shown in Sect. 3.1. This device is used to collect inertial data. The collected data is subject to filtering and feature extraction. Multiple ML-based classifiers are trained on the extracted features. The best performing ML model is then deployed on the hardware device by quantizing the ML model. The deployed ML model is then tested for accuracy.

3.1 Hardware Subsystem

The hardware construction of the device, and the data flow architecture is illustrated in Fig. 2.

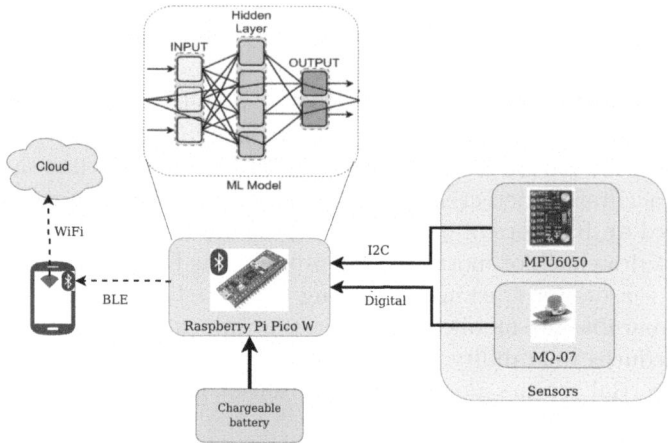

Fig. 2. Data flow for the proposed wearable device

The hardware subsystem of the device comprises of the following components. It is worth noting that this is a proof of concept device and the individual components can be replaced with lower power and smaller versions to achieve similar results.

- The proposed device is built around a Raspberry Pico W microcontroller board, which uses the ARM Cortex-M0+-based RP2040 microcontroller. The Pico W supports BLE and WiFi for communication. The device can also be built on low power devices like the Nordic Semiconductor's nrF52832 or Cypress PSoC 6 BLE., both of which support BLE for communication. The Pico W was only chosen to demonstrate the efficacy of the proposal.
- The sensor subsystem of the device comprises of a 6-axes inertial sensor - MPU6050, and a carbon monoxide sensor - MQ-7. The characteristics of the sensor are mentioned in Table 1. It is worth noting that we can use more miniaturized Carbon Monoxide sensors as well like the CJMCU-811.
- The power delivery mechanism is through a TP4056 battery charging module and is powered by a 1000mAh Li-Polymer battery.

The hardware device presented in Sect. 3.1 is attached to a wristband (as shown in Fig. 3 for data collection. It is to be noted that this is a proof of concept device. The final device can be custom fabricated as per the required dimensions.

Table 1. MPU-6050 (Accelerometer) and MQ-7 Gas Sensor Specifications

Specification	MPU-6050 (Accelerometer)	MQ-7 (CO Gas Sensor)
Supply Voltage	2.375 V to 3.46 V	5 V
Current Consumption	500 μA	< 350 mW
Measurement Range	± 2 g, ±4 g, ±8 g, ± 16 g	20 ppm to 2000 ppm
Response time	<1ms	<1 s
Operating Temperature	−40°C to +85°C	−10°C to 50°C
Humidity Range	N/A	10% to 95% RH

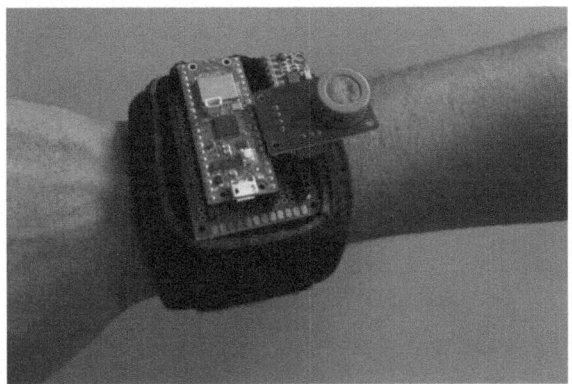

Fig. 3. The proposed wearable device

3.2 Software Subsystem

The software flow implemented on the designed wearable device is illustrated in Fig. 4. As mentioned in Fig. 2, the accelerometer data is used to train an ML model to classify a hand movement as smoking or non-smoking.

Since there are several actions that mimic the hand-to-mouth action involved in smoking, a carbon monoxide sensor is used to trigger the model. Only if the sensed carbon monoxide value is greater than a preset threshold, the ML model is triggered, thereby increasing selectivity. The threshold for CO was chosen to be 500 ppm as per literature [15]. For demonstrating the functionality of the device we use a preset threshold for the number of puffs which constitutes a cigarette. This value was set at 11, as per a study of human smoking patterns [29].

4 Building the ML Model

This section presents the details of the data collection process, followed by the features extracted from the data, and finally the training parameters.

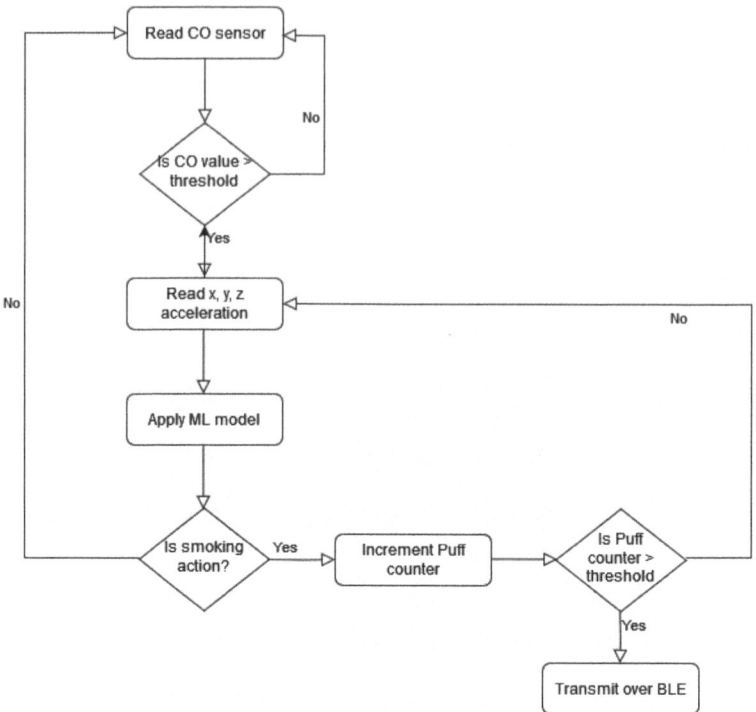

Fig. 4. Software flow for the proposed wearable device. CO threshold is set at 500 ppm [15]. Puff counter threshold is set at 11 [29]

4.1 Data Collection

Inertial data (x, y, and z acceleration) was collected from 10 individuals over 12 smoking sessions each, totaling 120 smoking sessions. The sampling rate was set at 33 Hz. The temporal graph of a smoking action spanning 5 s of a smoking action is shown in Fig. 5. The smoking pattern shows a clear pattern in y axis acceleration due to how the sensor was placed on the wrist. This pattern is to be recognized as a smoking action when the carbon monoxide sensor is triggered. Non-hand-to-mouth movement is more varied, a sample of which is shown in Fig. 6.

Data collection was done using Edge Impulse [9], which is an online suite to collect data, train machine learning models, and also quantize the models to deploy on constrained hardware systems like wearables. The software flow of the collection and training process is shown in Fig. 4.

4.2 Feature Extraction

From the collected data, 13 features, spectral and temporal, are extracted for each of the three acceleration axes, resulting in a total of 39 features. It is to be

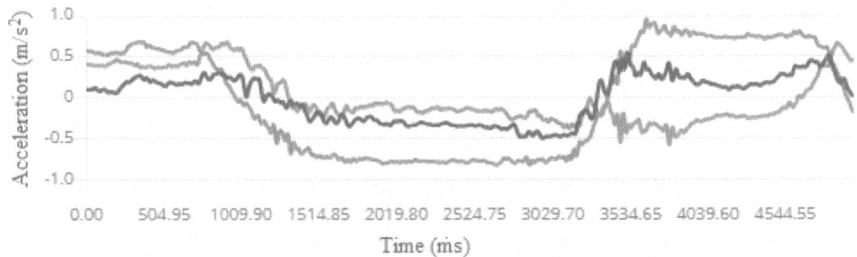

Fig. 5. X, Y, and Z temporal data for one smoking action

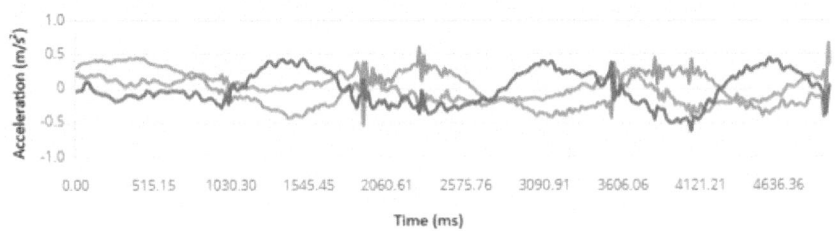

Fig. 6. X, Y, and Z temporal data for one non-smoking action

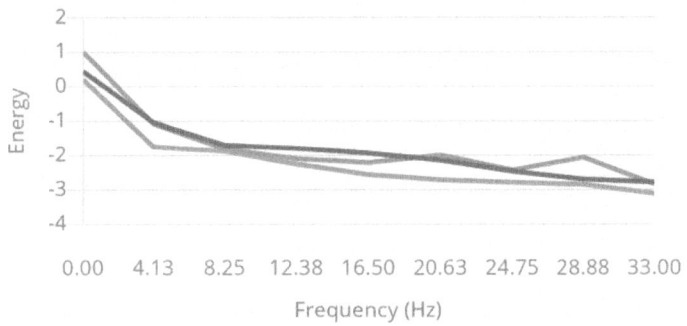

Fig. 7. Spectral Power Density for a smoking action

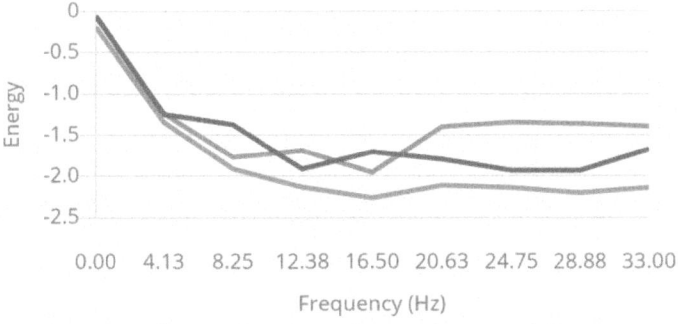

Fig. 8. Spectral Power Density for a non-smoking action

noted that although a 6-axis inertial sensor is used, the features are extracted only from the x, y, and z acceleration. This is because the yaw, pitch, and roll are significant only when there is a rotation about the axis of the sensor. The temporal features were *root mean square (RMS), skewness, kurtosis*. The spectral features were *spectral skewness* for the entire spectrum and *spectral power densities in 9 equidistant frequency intervals from 0–33* Hz *(sampling frequency)*. A sample of the spectral power graph is shown in Fig. 7. In comparison, the spectral power graph for a non-smoking action is shown in Fig. 8

4.3 Training Parameters

The extracted features were used to train four different ML models - Support Vector Machine (SVM), logistic regression, random classifier, and ridge classifier. It is to be noted that feature reduction was not explored in this paper. Each model is trained for 100 cycles and use 2 dense layers between the input and the output layers, as shown in Fig. 9. The training was done using 80% of the dataset collected. The learning rate is kept low to prevent overfitting. It is worth noting that the accuracy of the model may be increased on using other classifiers and different training parameters. However, the models chosen are sufficient to demonstrate the efficacy of tracking cigarette smoking using an accelerometer and a carbon monoxide sensor.

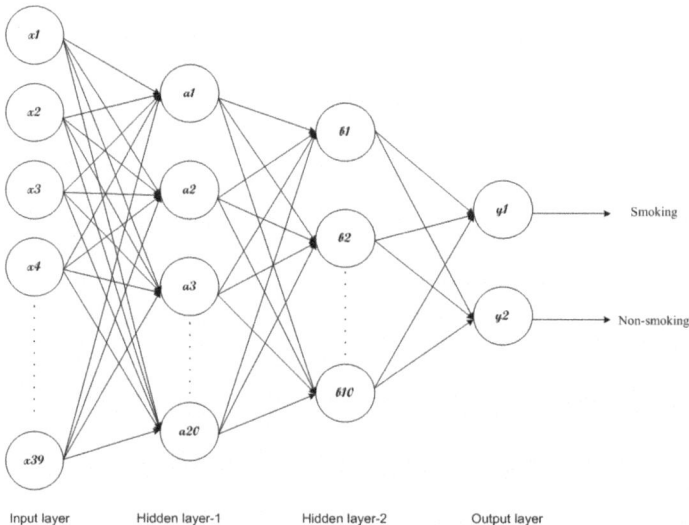

Fig. 9. The architecture of the ML models used

5 Results and Deployment

The accuracy of the trained ML models were evaluated and the results obtained are presented in Table 2. Please note that this accuracy is for the smoking action and not for the number of cigarettes smoked.

Table 2. Comparison of Classifier Performance

Parameters	Accuracy %	F1-score	
		Non-smoking	Smoking
Support Vector Machine	90.9	0.91	0.95
Logistic Regression	91	0.80	0.94
Random Forest Classifier	95.5	0.89	0.97
Ridge Classifier	93.8	0.91	0.96

From the results, it can be seen that the random forest classifier has the highest accuracy, and also the highest F1-score for classifying a smoking action. This was chosen for deployment on the wearable device.

Table 3. ML model deployment results

Parameter	Feature Extraction	Classifier	Total
Latency	52 ms	9 ms	61 ms
RAM	6.6 KB	1.1 KB	6.6 KB
Flash	-	15.4 KB	-
Accuracy	-	-	88%

The EON compiler which if part of the Edge Impulse suite was used to quantize the random forest classifier for deployment on the wearable device. All 32-bit floating point weights were converted to 8-bit integer weights so that lesser memory is required. The results of deployment are shown in Table 3.

Testing of the deployment was performed with 2 individuals over 10 individual smoking sessions. As shown, the quantization results in lower accuracy (88%) as compared with the accuracy of the non-quantized ML model (95.5%). It was observed that the ML model was activated only when the wearer was smoking i.e. the CO sensor value was above 500 ppm. This demonstrates the efficacy of the proposed device.

6 Conclusion and Future Scope

This paper introduces CigEst - a practical and reliable wearable device for monitoring cigarette smoking behaviour in real-world environments. The results indicate that integrating an inertial measurement unit (MPU6050) sensor with a carbon monoxide (MQ7) sensor provides improved outcomes for analyzing smoking behaviour compared to earlier studies on smoking detection. The ML model itself achieves a maximum accuracy of 95.5%, while the resource constrained ML model deployed on the wearable achieves a 88% accuracy. This accuracy can be further improved with training on a larger dataset, varying the training parameters, or using other ML algorithms.

References

1. Cress. http://www.borgwaldt.de/cms/borgwaldt-kc/produkte/rauchmaschinen/geraete-zur-rauchtopographie/cress-pocket.html
2. Smokerlyzer. http://www.bedfont.com/smokerlyzer
3. Ali, A.A., Hossain, S.M., Hovsepian, K., Rahman, M.M., Plarre, K., Kumar, S.: mPuff: automated detection of cigarette smoking puffs from respiration measurements. In: Proceedings of the 11th International Conference on Information Processing in Sensor Networks, pp. 269–280. IPSN 2012, Association for Computing Machinery, New York, NY, USA (2012). https://doi.org/10.1145/2185677.2185741
4. Bardot, S., et al.: One ring to rule them all: an empirical understanding of day-to-day smartring usage through in-situ diary study. Proc. ACM Interact. Mob. Wearable Ubiquitous Technol. **6**(3), 1–20 (2022)
5. Belsare, P., Senyurek, V.Y., Imtiaz, M.H., Tiffany, S.T., Sazonov, E.: DeepPuff: utilizing deep learning for smoking behavior identification in free-living environment. In: 2023 45th Annual International Conference of the IEEE Engineering in Medicine & Biology Society (EMBC), pp. 1–5. IEEE (2023)
6. Berry, K.M., Drew, J., Brady, P.J., Widome, R.: Impact of smoking cessation on household food security. Ann. Epidemiol. **79**, 49–55 (2023)
7. Charles, F.K.S., Krautter, G.R., Mariner, D.C.: Post-puff respiration measures on smokers of different tar yield cigarettes. Inhal. Toxicol. **21**, 712–718 (2009). https://api.semanticscholar.org/CorpusID:9170033
8. Cole, C.A., Janos, B., Anshari, D., Thrasher, J.F., Strayer, S., Valafar, H.: Recognition of smoking gesture using smart watch technology. arXiv preprint arXiv:2003.02735 (2020)
9. Hymel, S., et al.: Edge impulse: an MLOps platform for tiny machine learning (2023). https://arxiv.org/abs/2212.03332
10. Khalifa, O.O., Albagul, A., Khan, S., Islam, M.R., Usman, N.M.: Wireless smoke detection system. In: 2008 International Conference on Computer and Communication Engineering, pp. 409–413. IEEE (2008)
11. Kim, S., Lee, H., Kim, S., Lee, K.H., Yoo, S., Hong, J.E.: Effectiveness of a media literacy-based smoking prevention program in female adolescents. Public Health Nurs. **41**(3), 525–534 (2024)
12. Kong, G., et al.: Tobacco promotion restriction policies on social media (2024)
13. Liu, Y., Filippidis, F.T.: Tobacco market trends in 97 countries between 2007 and 2021. Tob. Induced Dis. **22**, 1–10 (2024)

14. Lopez-Meyer, P., Tiffany, S., Sazonov, E.: Identification of cigarette smoke inhalations from wearable sensor data using a support vector machine classifier. In: 2012 Annual International Conference of the IEEE Engineering in Medicine and Biology Society, pp. 4050–4053. IEEE (2012)
15. Pan, K.T., Leonardi, G.S., Ucci, M., Croxford, B.: Can exhaled carbon monoxide be used as a marker of exposure? A cross-sectional study in young adults. IJERPH **18**(22), 1–13 (2021). https://ideas.repec.org/a/gam/jijerp/v18y2021i22p11893-d677948.html
16. Panpaeng, S., Phanpeang, P., Metharak, E.: Cigarette smoke detectors for non-smoking areas in the building. In: 2018 22nd International Computer Science and Engineering Conference (ICSEC), pp. 1–4. IEEE (2018)
17. Parate, A., Chiu, M.C., Chadowitz, C., Ganesan, D., Kalogerakis, E.: RISQ: recognizing smoking gestures with inertial sensors on a wristband. In: Proceedings of the 12th Annual International Conference on Mobile Systems, Applications, and Services, pp. 149–161 (2014)
18. Pichandi, S., et al.: The effect of smoking on cancer-a review. Int. J. Biol. Med. Res. **2**(2), 593–602 (2011)
19. Raiff, B.R., Karataş, Ç., McClure, E.A., Pompili, D., Walls, T.A.: Laboratory validation of inertial body sensors to detect cigarette smoking arm movements. Electronics **3**(1), 87–110 (2014)
20. Sanger, J.B., Sitanayah, L., Kumenap, V.D.: Detection system for cigarette smoke. In: 2019 4th International Conference on Information Technology, Information Systems and Electrical Engineering (ICITISEE), pp. 145–149. IEEE (2019)
21. Senyurek, V.Y., Imtiaz, M.H., Belsare, P., Tiffany, S., Sazonov, E.: Smoking detection based on regularity analysis of hand to mouth gestures. Biomed. Signal Process. Control **51**, 106–112 (2019)
22. Shoaib, M., Scholten, H., Havinga, P.J., Incel, O.D.: A hierarchical lazy smoking detection algorithm using smartwatch sensors. In: 2016 IEEE 18th International Conference on e-Health Networking, Applications and Services (Healthcom), pp. 1–6. IEEE (2016)
23. Siersbaek, R., Kavanagh, P., Ford, J., Burke, S., Parker, S.: How and why do financial incentives contribute to helping people stop smoking? A realist review. BMC Public Health **24**(1), 500 (2024)
24. Sigmon, S.C., Patrick, M.E.: The use of financial incentives in promoting smoking cessation. Prev. Med. **55**, S24–S32 (2012)
25. Tang, Q.: Automated Detection of Puffing and Smoking with Wrist Accelerometers. Northeastern University (2014)
26. Triantafyllidis, A., et al.: Smartwatch interventions in healthcare: a systematic review of the literature. Int. J. Med. Inf. **190**, 105560 (2024)
27. Viscusi, W.K., Hakes, J.K.: Risk beliefs and smoking behavior. Econ. Inq. (2008). https://doi.org/10.1111/J.1465-7295.2007.00079.X
28. Wu, P., Hsieh, J.W., Cheng, J.C., Cheng, S.C., Tseng, S.Y.: Human smoking event detection using visual interaction clues. In: Proceedings of the 2010 20th International Conference on Pattern Recognition, pp. 4344–4347. ICPR 2010, IEEE Computer Society, USA (2010). https://doi.org/10.1109/ICPR.2010.1056
29. Zacny, J.P., Stitzer, M.L.: Human smoking patterns. Smoking Tobacco Control Monogr. **7**, 151–160 (1996)
30. Zaiedi, M.Z.M.: Air contaminants monitoring of carbon monoxide and hydrogen using standalone microcontroller based system for passive smoker. In: 2014 4th International Conference on Engineering Technology and Technopreneurship (ICE2T), pp. 171–176. IEEE (2014)

Digital Innovation for Individual Approach to Incorrect Spine Posture in Adolescents "NOVA-SPINE"

Gabriele Pontillo[1], Claudio Catalano[2(✉)], Viviana Andreozzi[2], Luca Maresca[3], and Sara Liguori[2]

[1] Università degli Studi di Firenze, 50127 Firenze, Italy
gabriele.pontillo@unifi.it
[2] Università degli Studi della Campania "L. Vanvitelli", 81100 Caserta, Italy
{claudio.catalano,viviana.andreozzi,sara.liguori}@unicampania.it
[3] Università degli Studi di Napoli "Federico II", 80121 Napoli, Italy
luca.maresca@unina.it

Abstract. Posture is a "habitual attitude" of an individual determined by the contraction of skeletal muscle groups that ensure a certain position of the body and its parts in space. Correct posture is determined by an ergonomically favorable state of neuro-musculoskeletal interaction to protect body structures from the appearance of deformities. Poor posture, with functional and symptomatic consequences, is common among adolescents in industrialized countries due to sedentary habits and significant changes in physical development and mental status, which trigger postural alterations such as hyperkyphosis and scoliosis. The current diagnostic approach to poor posture in this segment of the population is based mainly on visual inspection of the spine, which generally exhibits low-sensitivity features. At the same time, prevention of spinal deformities resulting from postural alterations through physical activity and self-correction of postural habits implemented during puberty has no scientific evidence and currently lacks adequate monitoring to show any benefits. The proposed research project, funded by the MUR under PRIN 2022 (D.D. No. 104/2022), proposes a new strategic model, which aims to potentially transform current diagnostic practices and provide a scientifically grounded approach to managing adolescent posture and long-term musculoskeletal health. Specifically, it introduces two different devices: NOVA-SPINE 1, a sensor-equipped diagnostic tool designed for enhanced precision, and NOVA-SPINE 2, a custom wearable device intended to support continuous postural management.

Keywords: Health Design · Posture Monitoring · Wearable Electronic Devices

1 Introduction

Poor posture is identified as an "abnormal bodily state" in which the individual's body is unable to ensure adequate stability in terms of balance and normal function of tissues and organs during the maintenance of upright posture [1]. This condition tends to occur more frequently during the growing period, involving up to 50% of adolescents, probably related to increased sedentary habits, significant changes in physical development and mental status, as well as biomechanical imbalance caused by rapid growth [2–4]. Clinical assessment of spinal alignment in adolescents is mainly based on visual observation of upright posture, in addition to the use of conventional screening methods such as Adam's anterior flexion test of the spine and measurement of spinal curves by radiographic scans. As for alternative techniques, such as photogrammetry, there is currently a lack of evidence to support their use in posture management [5] (Fig. 1).

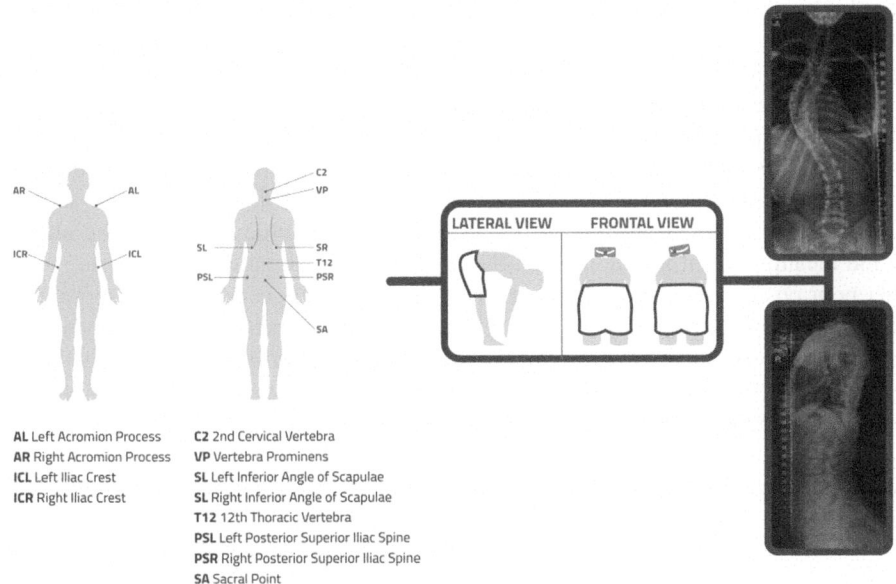

Fig. 1. Topic pathway related to current clinical practice for spine evaluation.

From a rehabilitative perspective, unlike scoliosis, the most common spinal deformity, there is no scientific evidence-based approach to managing poor posture in adolescents. For example, global postural retraining (GPR) is an individualized treatment that could reduce curve progression in patients with scoliosis [6]. However, further studies are needed to confirm the efficacy of this therapy and to more thoroughly understand its underlying biomechanical mechanisms [7]. To date, common clinical practice highlights the absence of a detailed and systematic assessment protocol for the diagnosis of poor posture and its management through specific and continuous physical activity. Therefore, early and comprehensive assessment of posture, accompanied by self-correction strategies and the practice of individualized therapeutic exercises, is essential to adequately address and treat postural problems in this population.

As of today, various attempts have been initiated in the field of medicine for different clinical application goals on posture assessment and monitoring, using electronic sensors and systems with advanced technology [8]. At the same time, wearable devices have sparked a growing interest in real-time posture monitoring, supporting the concept of the "quantified self" [9]. Wearable technology is a new interactive medium for collecting individual health data and providing immediate feedback, offering valuable information for clinicians to understand the correct protocol to follow and the effectiveness of that protocol over time [10]. Another advantage is that a properly developed device can also be useful for early diagnosis of diseases in the hospital setting, providing a numerical view of the patient's physical status, thus reducing waiting times for treatment and improving the effectiveness of the national health care system [11, 12]. Currently available devices can assess spinal posture with good accuracy in the clinical setting [13]. Motion tracking sensors, such as the Inertial Measurement Unit (IMU), have so far been the most popular technology in wearable systems used for the back. The 3D gyroscope, accelerometer, and magnetometer enable continuous and accurate 9-axis vector calculation of motion angles and accelerations. All current commercial devices detect back motion and, on the other hand, have several performance limitations [14].

However, the literature [15] offers investigations that rely solely on the presence of strain sensors, instead of microelectromechanical systems (MEMS) and particularly IMUs, to assess dynamic trunk movements during the day [16]. In addition, the sensory fusion of information from these different types of technology may also be able to provide meaningful information about the discomfort a patient experiences due to his or her poor posture. This is because, in addition to postural characteristics, appropriate sensor placement can provide a range of relevant information related to cardiorespiratory parameters, whose fluctuations are related to psychophysical stress [17, 18]. Although the literature on this application has been expanding for some years, most studies related to adolescent applications are limited to brief exploratory interactions with technologies designed for adults. The aim of this paper is to explore the current state of the art regarding wearable devices for the management of poor posture in pediatrics and to present our proposal within this context.

2 Main Findings on the Application of Wearable Devices for Posture Management in "Pediatric Populations"

Although the literature on this application has been expanding for several years, most studies related to apps for adolescents are limited to brief exploratory interactions with technologies designed for adults. To date, no tools, including wearables, have been validated for adolescents, particularly for the prevention, monitoring, and treatment of poor posture. Specifically, 4 articles peculiar to the type of study and target age group were selected from PubMed database:

1. Gal-Nadasan et al. [19] conducted a study using the Microsoft Kinect to detect scoliosis in 30 high school students. Overall posture was measured in an orthostatic position using the Microsoft Kinect, tracking key body points such as the hips and shoulders to form the postural data. The researchers found that the Kinect can be used to monitor changes in the spine and detect early signs of scoliosis and kyphosis, although it may not be as accurate as traditional screening methods. Active medical supervision is also critical to prevent further complications in individuals with existing problems.

2. In a 2021 study, Moreira et al. [20] developed and validated a mobile application called NLMeasurer for postural assessment. The application uses PoseNet, a computer vision and machine learning solution, to estimate human posture and identify anatomical points to calculate postural measurements. The study found that NLMeasurer agrees with validated biophotogrammetry software for postural measurements and demonstrated good inter- and intra-rater reliability. The use of surface markers on specific anatomical landmarks further improved the reliability of postural measurements.
3. Perimal et al. [21] collected accelerometer data from the Ocean Explorer game played by 60 children, revealing trends in posture changes, especially along the flexion and rotation axes. The study indicates that the game promotes stable vertical posture.
4. Cheung et al. [22] analyzed the subjective experience of 13 adolescents with mild scoliosis who participated in a postural training program with surface electromyography biofeedback. The program was found to improve symmetry of paraspinal muscle activities and reduce curve progression (Cobb's angle decreased by at least 5°) in 5 participants, while 8 participants showed changes in controlled Cobb's angle below 5° on radiographic examination. Those who benefited from the program reported improvements in posture, body appearance, muscle relaxation, reduction in pain and fatigue, self-confidence, and social functioning.

Following the analysis of the four scientific papers pertaining to the state of the art in testing innovative methods for surveying and postural assessment in adolescents, it was possible to outline the strengths and weaknesses of each case. Interestingly, the cases are marked by an increasingly advanced development of digital technologies, both for surveying parameters noninvasively and for a broader and more accurate reading of the data. The methodologies analyzed range from surveying postural data in the everyday setting, as in Gal-Nadasan et al., where the surveying is done via Kinect on a sample of students within the school environment, to a ludo-interactive method, as in Perimal et al., where the surveying part is done by simulating the movement of swimming within a video game. This also implies, a simplification in the task of data analysis by the physician who, in addition to a physical examination, can view the collected data for an optimal and more detailed analysis, such as in Moreira et al., 2021 where through the use of bio-photogrammetric techniques and Machine Learning technologies, it is possible to easily estimate the anatomical points of interest and extrapolate the data necessary for postural assessment.

The result of the literature review, however, showed that in addition to a greater and more accessible use of widely used digital technologies that give as output a wider range of data useful for postural assessments and diagnosis, what the cases examined have in common is the lack of a Design-Driven process, i.e., the absence of a specific, purpose-designed product that is not determined solely by technological sophistication, but by design factors that give the product peculiarities characteristic of Human Centered Design (HCD) and Life Centered Design (LCD) methodologies, such as ergonomics, usability, compliance, customization, accessibility and sustainability. Given the scarcity of data regarding the monitoring and diagnosis of posture in adolescents, we will refer to two studies conducted on adult populations to identify new or different methods for detecting postural abnormalities.

The study [23] conducted by researchers from the Schools of Mechatronic Systems & Engineering Science at Simon Fraser University (Metro Vancouver, Canada) describes the development of a wearable device based on textile sensors to monitor back movements, with the goal of preventing low back pain (LBP), which is the most common musculoskeletal disorder among healthcare workers due to poor posture and repetitive trunk movements. Traditionally, posture monitoring has been done through questionnaires, accelerometers, or optical sensing systems, but these have significant limitations, such as subjectivity of data, complexity in use, and the need for controlled environments. In response to these issues, the use of electronic textiles (E-textiles) offers an innovative and less invasive solution.

The developed system uses an inductive textile sensor created by sewing a copper wire into a stretchy fabric in a "zigzag" pattern that forms an inverted "T," promoting an increase in the inductance of the sensor, improving its sensitivity to fabric deformations caused by body movements. The zigzag configuration allows the tissue to stretch without damaging the sensoristics, improving the durability of the device during repetitive movements, and allowing it to specifically capture deformations in the lumbar region during forward bending resulting in reduced influence from other movements such as torsion or lateral bending. Sensor design was optimized using simulations conducted with Ansys software, which evaluated how different parameters of the zigzag pattern affect inductance with different pattern widths, showing that a smaller width offered the best compromise between sensitivity and comfort, being able to stretch up to 200% of the original length without breaking. The prototype was integrated into a tight-fitting bodysuit, chosen for its characteristics of comfort and adaptability to body movements, and placed over the lumbar region. The device was equipped with a wireless acquisition circuit, which included an inductance-to-digital converter (LDC1614), a microprocessor (Arduino Mini), and a Bluetooth module to transmit data to a smartphone application. The prototype was tested on a healthy participant performing a series of standardized movements, demonstrating that the sensor could effectively discriminate anterior bending movements, while lateral bending and torso twisting caused only slight changes in the inductance. During these tasks, the inductance of the sensor was recorded in real time and compared with angular data collected by two inertial measurement units (IMUs) positioned at the C7 and L5 vertebrae. Interference tests were also carried out with insignificant influences given by Wi-Fi signals and foreign metal objects.

While this study represents a significant contribution in the field of wearable devices for postural monitoring with a refinement of the smart-wearable concept and greater accuracy in parameter detection, it has some limitations. The test was conducted on only one healthy participant, which reduces the external validity of the results. Subjects with anthropometric variability or clinical conditions were not included, limiting the generalizability of the results. In addition, the study was not conducted in clinical or medical settings, and did not involve healthcare professionals, which hinders the possibility of transferring the results to real-world settings for clinical use and accurate diagnosis of any issues found by the findings. From a wearability perspective, the device is integrated into a fitted bodysuit that, although it optimizes wearability, is not modular, limiting the adaptability of the system to different sizes and body types. This makes it difficult to adapt the device to people with different sizes and body shapes, limiting its use to a specific target audience and compromising the accuracy of readings by the sensor system, especially during prolonged use.

Furthermore, the study conducted by a team of researchers affiliated with the Technical University of Munich (TUM) in Germany, discusses the use of a flexible wearable device for three-dimensional posture monitoring of the spine, with the goal of recognizing individuals' activities of daily living [24]. The detection of Activities of Daily Living (ADLs) is crucial for the diagnosis and management of diseases such as Alzheimer's, Parkinson's, and depression, as well as for monitoring the health status of the elderly. WHO has identified physical activity as a determinant of quality of life, and monitoring of spinal posture is particularly relevant to preventing and understanding the development of chronic low back pain (LBP). The device used is the FlexTail® [25], a strain sensor system 60 cm long and 2.5 cm wide, equipped with 25 sensor pairs distributed along the spine. The device is equipped with a three-axis accelerometer, a lithium-ion battery, internal memory, a microprocessor, and a Bluetooth and MicroUSB interface for data transmission to smartphones or computers. The device is worn with a tight-fitting T-shirt, equipped with a longitudinal pocket to keep the sensor stable but with a sufficient degree of freedom to follow the movements of the spine.

The study involved 30 subjects (22 males and 8 females) with an average age of 26.7 years, in good health and with no known pathologies. The activities analyzed were divided into three categories: static, dynamic and transitional. In total, 10 indoor activities, 4 outdoor activities, and 8 transitional states were identified. The activities were designed to represent various movements common in daily life, including bending, walking, running and position changes. Data were collected at a sampling rate of 5 Hz to ensure secure acquisition and reduce packet loss. The data was transferred to a computer via MicroUSB or via Bluetooth to a Raspberry Pi as a backup. Each dataset included 53 columns of data: 50 from the sensor strips and 3 from the accelerometer. For analysis, two graphical user interfaces (GUIs) were created to reduce the risk of errors in labeling the data. Transition tasks (TS) were labeled according to the duration of previous tasks and the visual difference between the transition signal and the other segments. For activity classification, three neural network models were implemented: LSTM (Long Short-Term Memory), CNN (Convolutional Neural Network), and a hybrid CNN-LSTM model. Each model was tested with time windows of two and ten seconds and with various data sets, including accelerometer, sensory strips and combinations of the two. The CNN model showed good accuracy for dynamic activities (walking and running) and static positions associated with lying down (RLD, supine and LLD), but had difficulty with bending and transition activities. The LSTM model achieved an overall accuracy of 80% with accelerometer data and 50% with sensory strip data. Combining the accelerometer and strip data improved the accuracy to 96%. The CNN-LSTM Hybrid model achieved an overall accuracy of 97%, showing improvements in bending tasks, but with difficulties in classifying transitions. The device was shown to be effective in monitoring daily activities and of potential utility in telemedicine for supervision of physical activities. However, the study has some limitations such as problems in positioning the device on taller subjects, with poor stability during complex movements such as bending backward. In addition, since the data surveying part is placed only on the spine, this does not facilitate a correct and comprehensive diagnosis through the different specific points placed on the torso, compromising an optimal evaluation by the specialist.

3 Our Proposal: The NOVA-SPINE Project

3.1 Goals and Description

In order to achieve advancement from the state of the art benchmark and improve those practices that are most closely related to the diagnosis and treatment of the pathological condition outlined, the NOVA-SPINE project will detect, record, and/or prevent poor posture and bad spinal habits during adolescence, through a tailored device, that will increase subjects' awareness, engagement, and compliance to treatment. The project proposes a new strategic model for the diagnosis, management, and monitoring of posture in growing subjects, using advanced technologies combined with the study and design of ergonomic and customized smart-wearable devices, divided into two kits:

- NOVA-SPINE 1: a wearable, sensorized diagnostic device capable of detecting the patient's postural data using a baropodometric platform and 3D scanning, in order to help the physician perform a meticulous assessment of posture and spinal dynamics. The collected data will be processed and viewed on a specific interface designed according to UI and UX criteria.
- NOVA-SPINE 2: a wearable device with integrated sensors to monitor physiological and postural parameters during exercise, promoting acceptability, compliance, and subject empowerment.

3.2 NOVA-SPINE KIT 1

In the first design phase, the NOVA-SPINE "KIT 1" device for measuring the morphology and dynamics of the spine will be developed. Integrated electronic sensors for measuring inertial parameters and strain and bending sensors will be adopted for this instrument. The first type of sensors consists of integrated circuits, typically identified as Magneto-Inertial Measurement Units (M-IMUs), in which data from accelerometers, gyroscopes and magnetometers are combined to reconstruct body-specific force, angular velocity and, with appropriate processing, body orientation. The solution will include custom stretchable variable resistors and piezoelectric sensors. The "KIT 1" device will be oriented to support the "medical examination," providing a compact tool for back posture assessment. Therefore, only direct measurement of body posture will be carried out. Three main aspects will be addressed at this stage:

- the selection of the most suitable M-IMU and strain sensors for "KIT 1";
- the development of the central circuit that can collect data from the sensors, process it and exchange it with an interface;
- the reduction of the size and power consumption of the central unit.

A sample of healthy subjects will be enlisted for preliminary testing, identifying specific landmarks of spinal posture chosen from current clinical methodologies [26], to acquire normative data with the NOVA-SPINE KIT 1 prototype. The data obtained from this evaluation will be archived in a database. The data obtained from this evaluation will be archived and analyzed, and a specific and simplified user interface will be created for the clinician, who will be able to extract posture parameters from the data obtained from the sensor system. For the prototyping of NOVA-SPINE KIT 1, the study of human factors and User-Centered Design (UCD) will be adopted as methods for observing, identifying, and analyzing user needs to determine strategies and design measures useful for the pursuit of clinical qualities in the field, such as increasing compliance, adherence, and participation in treatment, and thus clinical effectiveness. To ensure the required function, the NOVA-SPINE KIT 1 device will be developed through the use of design approaches and technologies such as additive manufacturing, going for a rigid and adjustable structure that incorporates its specific sensors to meet both the needs of detecting and assessing the degree of trunk and arm movement during ambulation and the needs of the field, making the device more comfortable and adaptable to individual users. The concept involves the use of a customizable t-shirt designed for the timely detection of the user's postural data, during the first observation phase. Through advanced Additive Manufacturing techniques, special surfaces for positioning the electronics and sensor part are 3D printed directly on the fabric and at the specific and delineated points of parameter detection. Using TPU as a flexible printing material, the surfaces adhere perfectly to the user's body while wearing the T-shirt, avoiding the compromise of ergonomics and parameter collection. For optimal positioning of the sensor and electronics component, the surface geometry printed on the fabric and composed of small cylinders (Male) allows the sensing sensors to be inserted inside specific covers (Female) that allow the interlocking and correct detection of postural data at specific points. A dedicated and user-friendly PC interface will be developed to support the clinician's assessment.

The testing phase will include young subjects, aged 11–21 years, enrolled and clinically evaluated at the outpatient clinic of Physical and Rehabilitation Medicine of the Azienda Ospedaliera Universitaria, University of Campania "Luigi Vanvitelli." According to the developmental stages of the American Academy of Child and Adolescent Psychiatry [27], subjects will be divided into 3 groups: early adolescence (11–14 years), middle adolescence (15–17 years), and late adolescence (18–21 years). During this examination, the clinician will use the NOVA-SPINE KIT 1 prototype to assess the subject's posture to obtain a detailed quantitative assessment of the alignment of the spine and its range of motion. In addition, each group in our population will perform gait analysis with NOVA-SPINE KIT 1 prototype applied, on a specific baropodometric platform (equipped with a load-sensing surface-force sensor array) and a 3D scanner to scan the subject, to obtain a comprehensive assessment of the degrees of movement of the trunk and arms. An investigation to test the tolerability of KIT 1 will be performed on the included population to further prototype with additive technologies an adaptable and adjustable device for different enrolled users.

3.3 NOVA-SPINE KIT 2

The second design phase will focus on the NOVA-SPINE "KIT 2" device. This is a specific wearable system that incorporates and integrates different sensors to continuously and simultaneously monitor: physiological parameters (e.g., respiration rate and pattern, heart rate and body temperature) using different sensor technologies; patient posture through distributed measurements on the posterior torso with sensors; physical activity (e.g., sitting, standing, walking, etc.) with inertial sensors; and patient environmental parameters (relative humidity and temperature). For "KIT 2," in addition to the M-IMU (ADXL355) and electromyography (EMG) sensors (Myoware© muscle sensor). Data coming from both IMU and EMG sensors will be collected by a central unit, implemented through microcontrollers, that will analyze through artificial intelligence (AI) the posture of the patient and will send data to a PC application, suitable for the medical evaluation of the patient. Since the goal of the "KIT 2" device is its wearability, the size of the control circuit will be minimized. For preliminary tests on the NOVA-SPINE KIT 2 prototype, a sample of healthy subjects will be enlisted, and a digital survey will be conducted, useful for the conformation of the three-dimensional model of the anatomical part to be treated, on which the customized device will be modeled. Following the same conception as Kit 1, NOVA-SPINE KIT 2 will be a wearable device customized to the individual user's anatomy, which will be fabricated through the use of several advanced digital techniques, such as 3D printing, direct-to-fabric 3D printing [28], and textile prototyping, that participate in the creation of a device that is innovative compared to the state-of-the-art reference. In addition, as a future development, KIT 2 will be equipped with an innovative posture feedback system that will give vibrotactile signals to the patient when he or she assumes an incorrect posture.

NOVA-SPINE KIT 2, through the identified approaches and technologies identified, will be lighter and more comfortable, breathable, smaller in size, and adapted to the user's body, thereby increasing compliance, psychological acceptance, participation, and, thus, treatment effectiveness, factors that as stated above determine those clinical qualities that can lead to innovation and progress over the state-of-the-art reference. After digital detection, each device will be assembled with integrated circuits and sensors and delivered to the subject. Our population will practice specific therapeutic exercises under the supervision of an experienced physical therapist at least three times a week for 3 months. At the end of the treatment, the data recorded by NOVA-SPINE KIT 2 prototype will be archived and a physician-specific user interface will be created. The safety (in terms of adverse outcomes) and tolerability (number of dropouts and withdrawals, size and weight satisfaction) of the device will be studied throughout the period. After these preliminary tests, prototyping of NOVA-SPINE KIT 2 prototype will be performed based on the feedback obtained.

The final testing phase will include the same sample used during testing of KIT 1 with a reevaluation, both clinical and using the NOVA-SPINE KIT 1 prototype, to avoid errors in posture assessment caused by the subject's potential growth over time. Within a maximum of 48 h after the assessment, the device will be delivered to the subject and a protocol of specific therapeutic exercises will be performed under the supervision of an experienced physical therapist at least three times a week for 3 months. At the end of the treatment, the data recorded by the NOVA-SPINE KIT 2 prototype will be archived and the physician will test the specific PC user interface for interpretation of the results. An investigation will be conducted to test the tolerability of KIT 2 to further prototype with additive technologies an adaptable and adjustable device for different enrolled users. To promote transparency in research, all data are available upon request.

4 Expected Outcomes and Challenges

As can be seen from the above analysis of the current state of the art, while many existing devices and studies are geared toward adults, NOVA-SPINE is specifically designed for adolescents, a population that faces unique challenges related to posture as they grow, representing an important innovation given the paucity of validated instruments for this group. With its dual-device design, NOVA-SPINE 1 for diagnosis and NOVA-SPINE 2 for continuous monitoring, it offers a synergistic approach that optimizes diagnostic accuracy and enables real-time postural monitoring through customized wearable devices designed to improve compliance and extended use by adolescents, an important aspect of early diagnosis and prevention. The integration of advanced sensors, including IMU and EMG sensors together with AI analysis of data, ensures detailed acquisition of postural parameters, while the customization of the NOVA-SPINE 2 wearable improves compliance and adaptability for adolescents, marking an advance over currently available standardized models.

NOVA-SPINE would be a key tool for screening and preventing poor posture among adolescents, providing useful solutions both for the objective quantitative assessment of this problem and, as an individualized non-invasive approach, to promote the subject's empowerment toward his or her physical and mental well-being. Wearing a device during an exercise program, such as comprehensive postural re-education, will allow for benefits during growth through the promotion of correct postural habits and counteracting sedentariness. It is expected to reduce the incidence of structural deformities of the spine, such as scoliosis, and increase the adoption of correct postural habits and active lifestyles among adolescents. In addition, given its customization, adaptability, and weight characteristics due to its soft and lightweight materials, we expect high comfort and tolerability of the device even while practicing the prescribed exercises. With this in mind, we also aim to reduce the dropout rates observed during conservative treatment of spinal deformities among adolescents. NOVA-SPINE will also improve knowledge of body posture while growing up by providing a huge collection of data on the spine of young subjects in a simple and intelligent way, reinforcing the concept of spinal deformity prevention by providing a deeper understanding of the effectiveness of comprehensive postural reeducation and self-correction as a preventive strategy in the management of poor posture and in the future, also for other common conditions that lead to poor spine posture such as low back pain.

For this project, there is a need to analyze the fabrics already on the market to evaluate the performance downstream of the integration of the sensor in the proposed garment. The specific shapes required for design purposes necessitate a specific optimization study to extract clean information from the sensitive elements due to movement artifacts caused by the biomechanics of the human body. Moreover, to further enhance the quality of the product, custom conductive ink with advanced screen-printing techniques will be employed. Lastly, it must be considered necessary to develop dedicated front-end electronics (central unit) to interrogate the sensors. In this scenario, the characterization of the sensing elements is crucial to correlate the strain and bending of the back of the patient to the ones provided as output from the sensing system, thus obtaining pivotal information to understand the back behavior. The EMG sensors selected for this application offer a high signal-to-noise ratio, ensuring greater reliability and precision. This is made possible by positioning the amplifier near the skin, significantly reducing noise and preserving signal integrity. Such a configuration enhances the accuracy of the collected data, which is critical for effectively training the AI system. By minimizing interference and capturing high-quality signals, these sensors contribute to the development of a more robust and efficient AI model, capable of delivering improved performance and outcomes in its intended application. This design choice is essential for ensuring optimal system functionality.

5 Conclusions

In conclusion, this review reveals substantial gaps in evaluation and treatment approaches for adolescent posture given by traditional methods, which can be addressed through the implementation of advanced technological medical devices designed to enhance diagnostic accuracy and reduce reliance on X-ray examinations, thus minimizing both radiation exposure and healthcare costs.

The miniaturization of electronic components and advancements in information technology have enabled the development of smart wearable devices that can play a transformative role in the E-Health landscape, especially as part of the ongoing Healthcare 4.0 movement.

In this scenario, among the different proposal described, NOVA-SPINE's dual diagnostic and therapeutic capabilities could not only enhance our understanding of biomechanical factors contributing to spinal misalignment but also promote early detection and treatment adherence among adolescents. By fostering healthy postural habits and enabling continuous monitoring of behaviors, NOVA-SPINE might bridge the gap between healthcare providers and young patients, facilitating a more engaged, patient-centered approach. This approach aligns with the biopsychosocial model of care, which is crucial for addressing the psychosocial challenges faced by adolescents dealing with spinal deformities, ultimately promoting their overall well-being and body image.

References

1. Dolphens, M., et al.: Sagittal standing posture and its association with spinal pain: a school-based epidemiological study of 1196 Flemish adolescents before age at peak height velocity. Spine **37**, 1657 (2012)
2. Sousa, A.S., Fonseca, I., Pichel, F., Amaral, T.F.: Effects of posture and body mass index on body girth assessment. Nutr. Clin. Pract. **31**(5), 690–694 (2016). https://doi.org/10.1177/0884533616629634. Epub 2016 Feb 17 PMID: 26888857
3. Duclos, M. : Effets de l'entraînement physique sur les fonctions endocrines [Effects of physical training on endocrine functions]. Ann. Endocrinol (Paris). **62**(1 Pt 1), 19–32 (2001). French. PMID: 11240404
4. Yang, L., Lu, X., Yan, B., Huang, Y.: Prevalence of incorrect posture among children and adolescents: finding from a large population-based study in China. iScience **23**(5), 101043 (2020). https://doi.org/10.1016/j.isci.2020.101043
5. Furlanetto, T.S., Sedrez, J.A., Candotti, C.T., Loss, J.F.: Photogrammetry as a tool for the postural evaluation of the spine: a systematic review. World J. Orthop. **7**(2), 136–148 (2016). https://doi.org/10.5312/wjo.v7.i2.136.PMID:26925386;PMCID:PMC4757659

6. Dupuis, S., Fortin, C., Caouette, C., et al.: Global postural re-education in pediatric idiopathic scoliosis: a biomechanical modeling and analysis of curve reduction during active and assisted self-correction. BMC Musculoskelet. Disord. **19**, 200 (2018)
7. Ma, K., Wang, C., Huang, Y., Wang, Y., Li, D., He, G.: The effects of physiotherapeutic scoliosis-specific exercise on idiopathic scoliosis in children and adolescents: a systematic review and meta-analysis. Physiotherapy **121**, 46–57 (2023). https://doi.org/10.1016/j.physio.2023.07.005
8. Wong, W.Y., Wong, M.S., Lo, K.H.: Clinical applications of sensors for human posture and movement analysis: a review. Prosthet. Orthot. Int. **31**(1), 62–75 (2007). https://doi.org/10.1080/03093640600983949. PMID: 17365886
9. Vijayan, V., Connolly, J.P., Condell, J., McKelvey, N., Gardiner, P.: Review of wearable devices and data collection considerations for connected health. Sensors **21**, 5589 (2021). https://doi.org/10.3390/s21165589
10. Ometov, A., Shubina, V., Klus, L., Skibińska, J., Saafi, S., Pascacio, P., et al.: A survey on wearable technology: history, state-of-the-art and current challenges. Comput. Netw. **193**, 108074 (2021). ISSN 1389-1286
11. Rechel, B., Wright, S., Nigel, E., Barrie, D., Martin, M.: Investing in hospitals of the future (2009)
12. Omachonu, V.K., Einspruch, N.G.: The Innovation Journal: The Public Sector Innovation Journal (2010)
13. Simpson, L., et al.: The role of wearables in spinal posture analysis: a systematic review. BMC Musculoskelet. Disord. **20**(1), 55 (2019). https://doi.org/10.1186/s12891-019-2430-6
14. Yoong, N.K.M., et al.: Commercial postural devices: a review. Sensors (Basel, Switzerland) **19**(23), 5128 (2019). https://doi.org/10.3390/s19235128
15. Mattmann, C., Amft, O., Harms, H., Tröster, G., Clemens, F.: Recognizing upper body postures using textile strain sensors. In: Proceedings - International Symposium on Wearable Computers, ISWC (2007)
16. Lee, I.M., Shiroma, E.J.: Using accelerometers to measure physical activity in large-scale epidemiological studies: Issues and challenges. Br. J. Sports Med. **48**, 197–201 (2014)
17. Butca, C.G., Suciu, G., Ochian, A., Fratu, O., Halunga, S.: Wearable sensors and cloud platform for monitoring environmental parameters in e-health applications. In: 2014 11th International Symposium on Electronics and Telecommunications, ISETC 2014-Conference Proceedings (2015)
18. Massaroni, C., et al.: Respiratory monitoring during physical activities with a multi-sensor smart garment and related algorithms. IEEE Sens. J. **20**(4), 2173–2180 (2019)
19. Gal-Nadasan, N., Gal-Nadasan, E.G., Stoicu-Tivadar, V., Poenaru, D.V., Popa-Andrei, D.: Measuring the negative impact of long sitting hours at high school students using the Microsoft Kinect. Stud. Health Technol. Inform. **236**, 383–388 (2017). PMID: 28508821
20. Moreira, R., et al.: A computer vision-based mobile tool for assessing human posture: a validation study. Comput. Methods Programs Biomed. **214**, 106565 (2022). https://doi.org/10.1016/j.cmpb.2021.106565. Epub 2021 Dec 4 PMID: 34936945
21. Perimal-Lewis, L., Light, J., Strobel, J.: UPRITE: promoting positive posture in children and adolescents. Stud. Health Technol. Inform. **29**(305), 495–498 (2023). https://doi.org/10.3233/SHTI230541. PMID: 37387075
22. Cheung, M.C., Yip, J., Law, D., Cheung, J.P.Y.: Surface electromyography (sEMG) biofeedback posture training improves the physical and mental health of early adolescents with mild scoliosis: a qualitative study. Digit Health. **24**(9), 20552076231203820 (2023). https://doi.org/10.1177/20552076231203820.PMID:37766906
23. García Patiño, A., Khoshnam, M., Menon, C.: Wearable device to monitor back movements using an inductive textile sensor. Sensors **20**, 905 (2020). https://doi.org/10.3390/s20030905

24. Haghi, M., Ershadi, A., Deserno, T.M.: Recognizing human activity of daily living using a flexible wearable for 3D spine pose tracking. Sensors **23**, 2066 (2023). https://doi.org/10.3390/s23042066
25. Minktek Homepage. https://minktec.com/technology/. Accessed 25 Sep 2024
26. Saltikov, J.B., Schreibe, S.: Innovations in Spinal Deformities and Postural Disorders (2017). https://doi.org/10.5772/intechopen.69575
27. Roscoe, B., et al.: Early, middle, and late adolescents' views on dating and factors influencing partner selection. Adolescence **22**(85), 59–68 (1987)
28. Pontillo, G., Langella, C.: Fluctuating Intelligence: Bioinspired 3D Printed Design on Textile. DIID—Disegno Industriale Ind. Des. **74**, 12–12 (2021)

Artificial Intelligence-Enabled Smart Glasses and Mobile Application for the Visually Impaired: Innovative Solutions in Wearable Health Technologies

Bekir Aksoy[✉] [iD], Mustafa Melikşah Özmen [iD], and Muzaffer Eylence [iD]

Faculty of Technology, Isparta University of Applied Sciences, Isparta, Turkey
bekiraksoy@isparta.edu.tr

Abstract. According to the reports of the World Health Organization (WHO), an average of 36 million people worldwide have completely lost their vision and 217 million people have moderate or severe visual impairment. Visually impaired individuals, who have an important place in society, face various difficulties in basic activities such as navigation, access to information, traffic safety, shopping or walking on the street in their daily lives. Safe movement of visually impaired individuals as pedestrians in traffic poses a great risk, especially due to the lack of audible signals and physical disabilities. Inability to read product information and price tags or not being able to follow the store layout during shopping are important problems that limit independence. Wearable health technologies developed for visually impaired individuals, especially artificial intelligence-supported smart glasses, offer innovative solutions to increase the independence of these individuals and improve their quality of life. Our study addresses the difficulties faced by visually impaired individuals and aims to overcome these difficulties with artificial intelligence-supported smart glasses. We will present the model we developed in order to obtain the best results by training artificial intelligence models with the natural data set we created. We will integrate the model we have created into the glasses and make it available to the user via a mobile application.

Keywords: Artificial intelligence · İmage processing · Mobile application

1 Introduction

Considering the world population, visually impaired individuals constitute an important segment of society. According to the 2019 report of the World Health Organization (WHO), 36 million people worldwide have completely lost their vision and 217 million people have moderate or severe visual impairment [1]. These data show that visually impaired people make up approximately 5% of the global population, and this rate reveals that a large segment of society faces serious limitations in basic daily activities.

Visually impaired individuals face various problems in their daily lives. In particular, basic needs such as shopping, moving safely in traffic as a pedestrian, and walking independently on the street pose serious obstacles for visually impaired individuals [2]. Difficulties such as not being able to read the information labels or prices of the products while shopping and not being able to follow the store layout restrict the opportunity of these individuals to shop independently [3]. Moving as a pedestrian in traffic carries a great risk due to the lack of audible signaling systems and physical obstacles, which brings about problems of safe crossing and navigation [4]. In addition, not being aware of physical obstacles or dangers while walking on the streets makes visually impaired individuals vulnerable to accidents [5].

The rapid development of technology offers new possibilities for solving such challenges. Especially in recent years, developments in the field of artificial intelligence have increased the potential of visually impaired individuals to overcome obstacles in their daily lives. Thanks to its ability to analyze large data sets, artificial intelligence allows visually impaired individuals to move more safely and independently by quickly detecting environmental variables and providing solutions tailored to the user's needs [6].

In this context, image processing techniques play a critical role for visually impaired individuals. Image processing is a technology that enables digital images to be analyzed and transformed into meaningful information, and forms the basis of many applications for the visually impaired. When combined with artificial intelligence algorithms, image processing technology; It offers effective solutions in many areas of use, such as recognizing product labels, detecting and guiding physical obstacles [7]. For example, during a shopping session, artificial intelligence-supported smart glasses can read the barcodes or labels of products through cameras and present this information to the user as voice feedback [8]. Similarly, smart glasses for individuals moving in traffic or on foot can detect surrounding vehicles, pedestrian crossings or potential dangers, allowing the user to move safely [9].

The fact that artificial intelligence and image processing offer such powerful solutions shows the potential of smart devices to be developed for visually impaired individuals to increase their independence and improve their quality of life. In this study, an artificial intelligence-supported smart glasses solution will be discussed to solve the daily problems faced by visually impaired individuals. This solution, developed to overcome the difficulties encountered during shopping, traffic safety and walking on foot, aims to increase the independence of visually impaired people. In this context, the aim of the developed artificial intelligence models is to detect environmental factors quickly and accurately and provide feedback to the user. In particular, data sets and model training processes in which image processing techniques are used will be detailed and findings regarding the performance of the developed system will be presented.

2 Material and Methods

2.1 Material

2.1.1 Dataset

A unique dataset has been created for the detection and real-time recognition of tactile walking paths for visually impaired individuals on pedestrian walkways. Within the scope of this study, a total of 2,300 images, captured under different road types and various weather conditions, were collected using an iPhone 11 device. The high resolution of the images enabled detailed analysis of the paths and the guide lines that indicate walking directions. These images, collected for the training of an artificial intelligence-based model, underwent preprocessing steps as a priority. These steps included resizing the images to 224×224 pixels and converting them to grayscale. The grayscale conversion reduced the data size, facilitating faster and more effective model training.

During the preprocessing phase to make the images suitable for artificial intelligence algorithms, various filtering techniques were employed to eliminate noise and unwanted elements. Specifically, the Gaussian filtering method was applied to reduce noise, with the goal of enabling clearer image processing. Additionally, normalization was performed to ensure the images had consistent scale and distribution, which played a crucial role in accelerating the model's learning process. After these stages, each image in the dataset was meticulously annotated in terms of the regions containing tactile walking paths for the visually impaired and their structural features. The annotation process was conducted in detail to enhance the model's accuracy, clearly indicating the presence, direction, and condition of the tactile walking paths in each image.

The dataset created in this study provides a valuable resource for the development of artificial intelligence-based tactile walking path detection systems for visually impaired individuals. The collected data spans a wide range of environmental conditions and various road structures, simulating real-world scenarios. In this way, the general validity and applicability of the developed system can be tested, with the aim of ensuring the safe navigation of visually impaired individuals on pedestrian walkways and enhancing traffic safety.

2.1.2 Convolutional Neural Network

Convolutional Neural Networks (CNNs) have witnessed significant advancements in recent years, particularly with applications in image processing, object detection, and natural language processing. In 2024, novel research has focused on improving the efficiency and accuracy of CNNs by optimizing architectures, reducing computational complexity, and enhancing transfer learning techniques. One of the key developments has been the integration of hybrid models, which combine CNNs with other neural network frameworks, such as transformers, to enhance the contextual understanding of images and sequences. Studies have demonstrated that these hybrid models outperform traditional CNNs in tasks like object detection and segmentation, providing better accuracy with fewer parameters [10].

Furthermore, the incorporation of pruning methods has contributed to reducing the memory footprint of CNNs, particularly in resource-constrained environments, without sacrificing accuracy. Researchers have proposed new pruning techniques that dynamically adjust during training, allowing CNNs to retain essential features while minimizing computational costs [11]. Another critical area of exploration is the application of CNNs in 3D data analysis, where advancements in volumetric CNN architectures have enabled more accurate analysis of 3D medical images and point cloud data [12].

Moreover, recent work on attention mechanisms within CNN architectures has shown that adding spatial and channel attention modules can improve feature selection processes, enhancing performance in complex image classification tasks [13]. These mechanisms allow CNNs to focus on the most critical regions in an image, which is particularly useful in tasks like facial recognition and object localization [14]. Additionally, research has highlighted the importance of data augmentation strategies in improving the robustness of CNN models against adversarial attacks, with new augmentation techniques being developed to counteract common perturbations in input data [15].

CNN-based models are also being adapted for multimodal data processing, with successful implementations in combining visual and textual information for tasks like image captioning and video understanding [16]. Lastly, the application of explainable artificial intelligence (XAI) techniques to CNNs has gained momentum, aiming to enhance the interpretability of these models in high-stakes domains like healthcare and autonomous driving [17, 18]. The improvements in explainability ensure that CNN models can be audited, making them more trustworthy and transparent [19].

2.1.3 Yolo v8

YOLOv8 (You Only Look Once, version 8) represents a substantial advancement in real-time object detection frameworks, building on the foundation of its predecessors by improving accuracy, speed, and flexibility. One of the notable innovations in YOLOv8 is its ability to balance precision and computational efficiency through a more refined architecture that incorporates better feature extraction and a deeper network design. Research in 2024 has focused on optimizing YOLOv8 for deployment in various edge devices, such as drones, autonomous vehicles, and mobile phones, where processing power is limited [20].

Incorporating advanced attention mechanisms, such as the Convolutional Block Attention Module (CBAM), YOLOv8 enhances the model's ability to focus on critical regions of an image while ignoring irrelevant background noise. This results in improved detection performance, particularly in scenarios with complex backgrounds or small objects [21]. Another significant improvement is the model's flexibility, allowing it to perform not just object detection, but also segmentation and keypoint estimation within the same framework. Studies have shown YOLOv8's performance to be on par with specialized segmentation models, further widening its application scope [22].

A key area of research in 2024 has been the application of YOLOv8 in real-time aerial image analysis, where its lightweight architecture has been utilized for detecting vehicles, pedestrians, and infrastructure anomalies from UAVs with great accuracy [23]. Furthermore, new training paradigms involving knowledge distillation and transfer learning have enabled YOLOv8 to retain high accuracy even when trained on smaller, domain-specific datasets [24]. This makes it particularly effective for custom object detection tasks in industrial settings, where labeled data may be limited.

YOLOv8 also benefits from improved loss functions, such as the introduction of a hybrid IoU loss, which helps in achieving more precise bounding box predictions, reducing localization errors during object detection [25]. This has been particularly beneficial in detecting overlapping or occluded objects, which is a known challenge in dense environments like urban traffic or crowded public spaces [26]. Additionally, YOLOv8's deployment in the context of smart city infrastructure, including traffic management and surveillance systems, has shown promising results, with enhanced real-time processing capabilities and accurate anomaly detection [27, 28].

Finally, the explainability of YOLOv8 has been a focus of recent studies, with researchers integrating explainable AI (XAI) techniques to make the decision-making process of the model more transparent, especially in critical applications like autonomous driving and public safety [29].

2.1.4 MobileNet V3

MobileNetV3, the latest iteration in the MobileNet series, continues to push the boundaries of efficient deep learning models, particularly for mobile and edge computing devices. This architecture leverages several key innovations to balance computational cost and accuracy, making it a popular choice for applications like real-time image classification and object detection on resource-constrained devices. A major advancement in MobileNetV3 is the use of the "squeeze-and-excitation" (SE) blocks, which allow the model to recalibrate channel-wise feature responses, leading to more accurate representations [30]. These blocks, combined with the efficient use of depthwise separable convolutions, significantly reduce the number of parameters and operations without compromising performance.

In 2024, research has highlighted the use of MobileNetV3 in various edge AI tasks, including its successful implementation in mobile healthcare applications, where real-time data processing is crucial. Studies demonstrate that MobileNetV3's lightweight architecture enables seamless integration into wearable devices, providing high-quality diagnostics in scenarios such as real-time medical image analysis [31]. Additionally, MobileNetV3 has been optimized for tasks involving facial recognition, where it outperforms larger models in terms of speed and accuracy on mobile devices [32].

A key area of focus in recent research is the combination of MobileNetV3 with quantization techniques to further reduce model size and power consumption, which is critical for deploying AI models in IoT devices and smart sensors [33]. Researchers have also explored the application of MobileNetV3 in video understanding tasks, with novel adaptations of the model allowing it to process video frames more efficiently, making it suitable for real-time applications like video surveillance and gesture recognition [34].

Furthermore, MobileNetV3 has been integrated into autonomous vehicle systems, where its compact size and low latency enable real-time object detection and lane tracking, even in complex urban environments [35]. The model's ability to maintain high accuracy with fewer resources makes it ideal for deployment in embedded systems, where computational power and energy consumption are primary concerns [36].

Recent studies have also explored the explainability of MobileNetV3, using explainable AI (XAI) methods to better understand the decision-making processes in real-time mobile applications. This has led to more interpretable AI systems, particularly in critical areas like healthcare and autonomous navigation [37].

2.1.5 Performance Evaluation Metrics

In artificial intelligence applications, model performance evaluation metrics such as accuracy, precision, recall, and F1 score are crucial for understanding the effectiveness and generalization capabilities of models. Accuracy measures the proportion of correctly classified instances among the total instances and is useful for balanced datasets. However, in imbalanced datasets, accuracy may be misleading, as it could still yield a high value despite the model failing to capture the minority class effectively [38].

Precision, on the other hand, measures the ratio of true positive predictions to the total positive predictions. This metric is particularly important in scenarios where minimizing false positives is critical, such as in medical diagnostics, where unnecessary treatments could have serious consequences [39]. Recall quantifies how well the model identifies all relevant instances, focusing on minimizing false negatives. For instance, in disease detection systems, high recall is essential to ensure that all cases are correctly identified [40].

F1 score, the harmonic mean of precision and recall, balances these two metrics to give a more comprehensive view of model performance. This metric is particularly valuable when dealing with imbalanced datasets, as it accounts for both types of classification errors (false positives and false negatives) [41].

In more complex applications, metrics like the Receiver Operating Characteristic (ROC) curve and Area Under the Curve (AUC) are also employed. The ROC curve visually represents the trade-offs between true positive and false positive rates as the classification threshold is varied, while AUC provides a single scalar value summarizing the overall performance. A high AUC indicates that the model achieves a good balance between precision and recall [42].

Thus, evaluating model performance based solely on accuracy can be misleading, especially in imbalanced datasets. A more holistic evaluation should consider metrics like precision, recall, F1 score, and AUC to provide a reliable understanding of model behavior in real-world scenarios [43].

2.1.6 Mobile Application

Flutter, a popular open-source framework for mobile application development, has gained significant traction for its ability to create high-performance, natively compiled applications across multiple platforms. Its flexibility and ease of use have made it an attractive option for integrating artificial intelligence (AI) capabilities within mobile applications. In recent years, combining Flutter with AI technologies has opened up new possibilities for developing intelligent, responsive apps. One of the key benefits of using Flutter in AI-driven applications is its ability to handle real-time data processing efficiently, making it suitable for AI tasks like image recognition, natural language processing, and predictive analytics [44].

With the integration of pre-trained machine learning models through frameworks such as TensorFlow Lite and PyTorch Mobile, developers can easily embed AI functionalities into Flutter applications. This allows for offline processing of AI tasks, enabling applications to function without an internet connection, which is particularly useful in areas with limited connectivity [45]. Additionally, Flutter's support for integrating with cloud-based AI services, such as Google's ML Kit and Firebase, further expands its capabilities by allowing real-time model updates and improved performance in tasks like facial recognition, object detection, and sentiment analysis [46].

One of the critical aspects of combining Flutter with AI is its role in enhancing user experience. AI models embedded within Flutter applications can learn from user interactions, adapting the app's behavior to provide personalized services. This is particularly useful in mobile health applications, where AI algorithms can process sensor data in real-time to provide instant feedback on health metrics like heart rate or activity levels [47]. Furthermore, AI-powered Flutter apps have been applied in fields such as autonomous driving and smart home systems, where real-time decision-making and responsiveness are essential [48].

Overall, Flutter's versatility and its seamless integration with AI tools make it a powerful framework for developing intelligent mobile applications. The ability to create cross-platform apps with AI functionalities has revolutionized how developers approach mobile app development, particularly in areas requiring real-time data analysis and personalized user experiences [49].

2.2 Method

First, a dataset was created to detect tactile walking paths for visually impaired individuals on pedestrian walkways. This dataset consists of 2,300 images captured under various road types and weather conditions using an iPhone 11. The high-resolution images were collected to analyze the tactile guidelines that indicate walking directions in detail.

After the dataset was created, the images were processed to make them suitable for the artificial intelligence (AI) model. These preprocessing steps included resizing the images to 224x224 pixels, converting them to grayscale, and reducing noise using Gaussian filtering. Additionally, normalization was applied to ensure consistent data handling. Each image was meticulously annotated based on the presence, direction, and condition of the tactile paths.

In the final stage, a model was trained using a Convolutional Neural Network (CNN) architecture. CNN layers extracted necessary features from the images to identify the tactile walking paths. The model training was carried out using 80% of the dataset for training and 20% for validation. The model's performance was tested and optimized using the validation set.

FINDINGS

This study focused on AI-powered smart glasses and mobile application solutions designed to improve the quality of life for visually impaired individuals. By addressing the challenges faced in daily activities such as traffic safety, shopping, and walking, the proposed technology aims to enhance the independence of visually impaired individuals.

The deep learning models trained with the dataset used in our study allowed for the detection of environmental obstacles and factors, ensuring safer movement for users.

Notably, the YOLO v8 and MobileNet V3 deep learning models achieved high accuracy rates. Table 1 below summarizes the performance of these models.

Table 1. Performance evaluation metrics

Model	Accuracy	Precision	Recall	F1 Score
CNN (Custom Model)	0.9245	0.856101	0.918368	0.886142
MobileNet V3	0.9122	0.858656	0.945679	0.900069
YOLO V8	0.9154	0.888676	0.859841	0.874021

As shown in Table 1, both YOLO v8 and MobileNet V3 models exhibited excellent performance. YOLO v8 excelled in real-time object detection and environmental analysis, making it especially useful for traffic safety and obstacle detection. Meanwhile, MobileNet V3 stood out with its low resource consumption and high efficiency, making it ideal for use on mobile devices.

The smart glasses, equipped with these AI models, provided significant benefits in daily activities. Users were able to read product labels while shopping, move safely in traffic, and detect obstacles on the streets. The AI-powered glasses provided users with audio feedback, ensuring a more independent lifestyle. The images below illustrate practical applications of the models trained with the dataset.

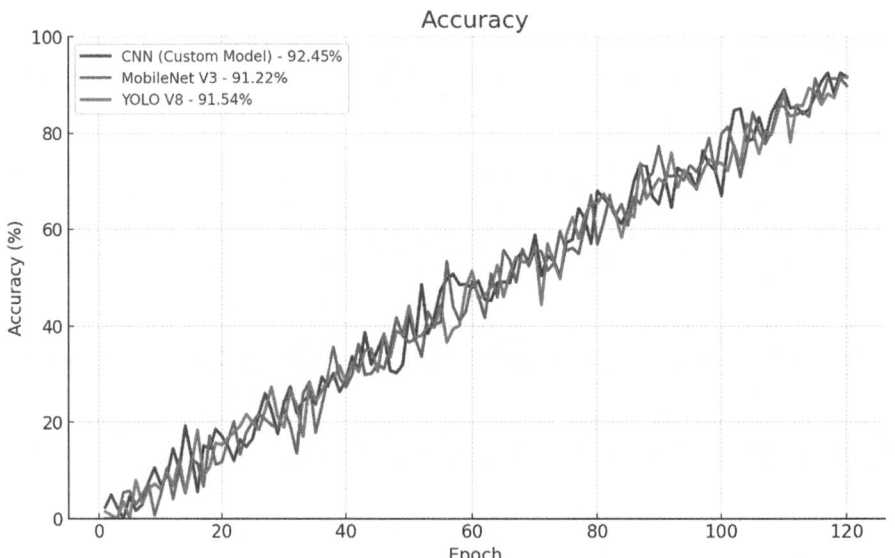

Fig. 1. Accuracy graph

Figure 1 shows the accuracy performance during the training process for three different deep learning models: CNN Custom Model, MobileNet V3, and YOLO V8. The graph allows us to observe how the accuracy of each model evolves during training and compare their final accuracy rates.

In Fig. 1, the CNN Custom Model (blue line) shows a more stable increase in accuracy compared to the other models, reaching the highest performance with an accuracy rate of 92.45%. From the beginning of the training process, the accuracy steadily increases, and although there are some fluctuations, this model consistently maintains the highest accuracy.

The MobileNet V3 (green line) achieves an accuracy of 91.22%. Although there are slight fluctuations compared to the other models, the overall accuracy remains high. Optimized for mobile device usage, MobileNet V3 provides a reasonable accuracy rate despite its low computational cost.

The YOLO V8 (red line) reaches an accuracy of 91.54%, which is very close to the other two models. Initially, YOLO V8 follows a similar trend to the other models, but towards the end of the training process, it shows slightly lower performance, though it still reaches a high accuracy level overall. YOLO V8 stands out as an ideal option for real-time object detection and environmental analysis.

In conclusion, all three models achieved high accuracy rates throughout the training process, with the CNN Custom Model performing the best. However, MobileNet V3 and YOLO V8 models also show great potential for practical use due to their lower computational costs and suitability for mobile and real-time applications.

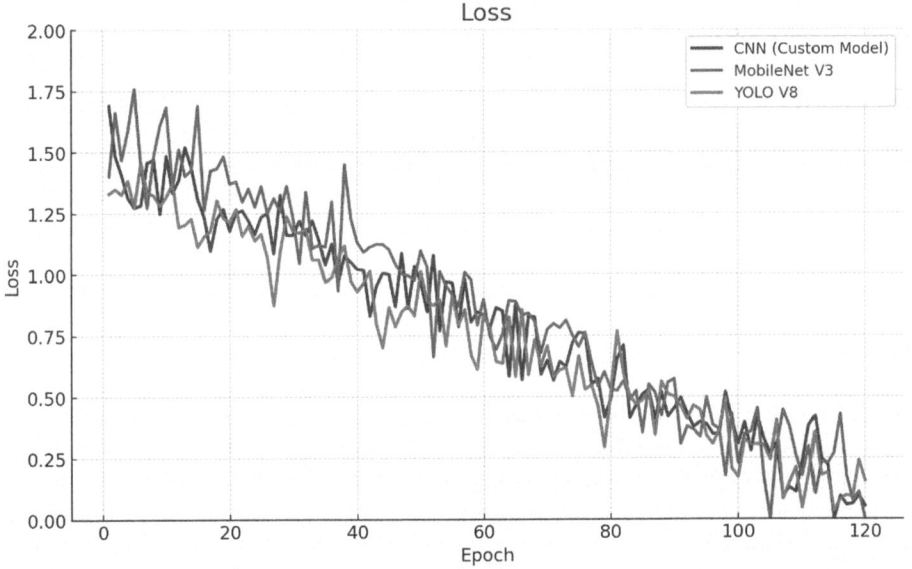

Fig. 2. Loss graph

Figure 2 illustrates the loss performance of three different deep learning models (CNN Custom Model, MobileNet V3, and YOLO V8) throughout the training process. Loss refers to the error between the predicted values and the actual values, with a lower loss indicating a better performing model.

In Fig. 2, the CNN Custom Model (blue line) demonstrates a consistent decrease in loss over time, following a relatively steady path with minimal spikes. By the end of the training process, the loss has decreased significantly, indicating that the model has effectively learned to minimize errors during training.

The MobileNet V3 model (green line) initially shows higher volatility in the loss values, especially during the first half of the training. However, the loss gradually decreases and converges toward a lower value, although it fluctuates more compared to the other models. This suggests that MobileNet V3 required more adjustments during training but still managed to achieve a reasonable reduction in loss by the end.

The YOLO V8 model (red line) starts with a slightly lower loss than the other models and consistently maintains a smoother trajectory, with fewer fluctuations. By the end of the training process, YOLO V8 exhibits the lowest overall loss, indicating that it has learned more efficiently and effectively minimized prediction errors.

Overall, Fig. 2 highlights the progression of all three models during training. The CNN Custom Model and YOLO V8 show more stable learning patterns, with YOLO V8 achieving the lowest final loss. MobileNet V3, while more erratic in the early stages, still demonstrates improvement, though with slightly higher final loss values.

3 Conclusion

In conclusion, this study presents innovative solutions in wearable health technology aimed at improving the quality of life for visually impaired individuals. The integration of artificial intelligence (AI)-supported smart glasses and mobile applications demonstrates significant potential in overcoming the challenges faced by these individuals in daily activities such as navigating traffic, shopping, and independent walking. By leveraging advanced image processing techniques and deep learning models like YOLO v8 and MobileNet V3, the developed system effectively detects environmental obstacles and provides real-time feedback to users, significantly enhancing their independence and safety.

The performance of the AI models, as evidenced by the high accuracy rates achieved in this study, showcases the effectiveness of utilizing AI in wearable devices. YOLO v8's superior real-time object detection capabilities and MobileNet V3's efficiency in mobile platforms contribute to making the proposed system not only accurate but also practical for everyday use. As technology continues to evolve, the deployment of such AI-powered systems could lead to broader applications and further improvements in accessibility for visually impaired individuals.

Future work could focus on expanding the dataset to cover a wider range of environments and incorporating additional features into the smart glasses, such as integrating speech recognition for enhanced interaction. Additionally, exploring other AI architectures could yield even more refined solutions, further increasing the system's adaptability and accuracy in diverse scenarios.

References

1. World Health Organization. World Report on Vision. World Health Organization. Author, F., Author, S.: Title of a proceedings paper. In: Editor, F., Editor, S. (eds.) CONFERENCE 2016, LNCS, vol. 9999, pp. 1–13. Springer (2019)
2. Wahl, H.W., Oswald, F., Zimprich, D.: Everyday competence in visually impaired older adults: a case for person-environment perspectives. Gerontologist **39**(2), 140–149 (1999)
3. Erdoğan, S., Yılmaz, H.: Görme Engellilerin Alışverişte Yaşadığı Problemler ve Teknolojik Çözümler. Teknoloji ve Toplum Araştırmaları Dergisi **5**(2), 89–102 (2018)
4. Yıldırım, A.: Görme Engelliler İçin Trafik Güvenliği ve Sesli Sinyalizasyon Sistemlerinin Önemi. Ulaşım ve Güvenlik Dergisi **9**(1), 17–29 (2021)
5. Demir, B., Aydın, N.: Görme Engellilerde Yaya Olarak Hareket Ederken Karşılaşılan Riskler. Engellilik Araştırmaları Dergisi **6**(4), 103–116 (2020)
6. Zhang, L., Zhang, L.: Artificial intelligence for remote sensing data analysis: a review of challenges and opportunities. IEEE Geosci. Remote Sens. Mag. **10**(2), 270–294 (2022)
7. Zhang, X., Dahu, W.: Application of artificial intelligence algorithms in image processing. J. Vis. Commun. Image Represent. **61**, 42–49 (2019)
8. Demir, T., Kılıç, O.: Akıllı Gözlük Teknolojilerinin Görme Engellilere Sağladığı Faydalar. Yapay Zeka Teknolojileri Dergisi **8**(1), 66–82 (2021)
9. Karadeniz, Y.: Trafikte Görme Engelliler İçin Geliştirilen Akıllı Teknolojilerin Değerlendirilmesi. Ulaşım Teknolojileri Dergisi **7**(3), 48–59 (2020)
10. Zhang, X., Li, Y., Wu, J.: Hybrid CNN-transformer architectures for enhanced image classification. IEEE Trans. Neural Netw. Learn. Syst. (2024)
11. Chen, T., Liu, M., & Zhao, P. (2024). Dynamic pruning for efficient CNNs: A review and future directions. Journal of Machine Learning Research
12. Wang, H., Singh, R.: Volumetric CNNs for medical 3D image segmentation: a comparative study. Med. Image Anal. (2024)
13. Zhao, X., Sun, Y., & Lin, F. (2024). Attention-enhanced CNN architectures for object detection. Computer Vision and Image Understanding
14. Kim, D., Park, S.: Channel attention mechanisms in CNNs for robust facial recognition. Pattern Recogn. Lett. (2024)
15. Xu, Z., Wang, L.: Data augmentation techniques for CNNs: enhancing robustness against adversarial attacks. IEEE Access (2024)
16. Gao, Y., Zhu, C.: Multimodal CNNs for image and text-based video understanding. Pattern Recogn. (2024)
17. Li, Q., Luo, J.: Towards explainable CNNs: XAI methods and applications in healthcare. J. Artif. Intell. Res. (2024)
18. Johnson, M., Patel, V.: Explainable CNNs in autonomous driving: Challenges and solutions. IEEE Trans. Auton. Syst. (2024)
19. Sun, K., Zhang, Z.: Enhancing the interpretability of CNNs with attention-based explanations. Expert Syst. Appl. (2024)
20. Wang, T., Zhao, J., Liu, Q.: Optimizing YOLOv8 for edge computing: applications in real-time UAV detection. J. Real-Time Image Process. (2024)
21. Huang, L., & Shen, Y. (2024). Enhanced object detection using attention modules in YOLOv8. Pattern Recognition Letters
22. Chen, F., Zhang, K.: YOLOv8: a unified framework for detection, segmentation, and keypoint estimation. Comput. Vis. Image Underst. (2024)
23. Li, J., Wu, H.: Real-time aerial surveillance with YOLOv8: applications in traffic management. IEEE Trans. Geosci. Remote Sens. (2024)

24. Sun, Y., Wei, R.: Transfer learning in YOLOv8: a case study in industrial defect detection. J. Mach. Learn. Res. (2024)
25. Zhao, Y., He, J.: Bounding box refinement in YOLOv8 with hybrid IoU loss. IEEE Trans. Image Process. (2024)
26. Lin, D., Xu, Z.: Overcoming occlusion in object detection: a comparison of YOLOv8 and other state-of-the-art models. Int. J. Comput. Vis. (2024)
27. Lee, S., Park, M.: YOLOv8 for smart city surveillance: real-time object detection and tracking. Sensors (2024)
28. Kim, H., Choi, J.: Anomaly detection in urban environments using YOLOv8. Expert Syst. Appl. (2024)
29. Zhang, F., Liu, S.: Explainable YOLOv8: improving transparency in object detection for autonomous systems. J. Artif. Intell. Res. (2024)
30. Liu, X., Zhao, W.: Channel recalibration with SE blocks in MobileNetV3 for efficient image classification. IEEE Trans. Neural Netw. Learn. Syst. (2024)
31. Wang, T., Sun, L.: MobileNetV3 for real-time medical image analysis on mobile devices. J. Biomed. Inf. (2024)
32. Chen, F., Liu, Z.: Lightweight facial recognition with MobileNetV3: a mobile-friendly approach. Pattern Recogn. (2024)
33. Zhang, J., Wang, Y.: Quantization-aware training of MobileNetV3 for edge AI applications. IEEE Trans. Image Process. (2024)
34. Gao, H., Li, M.: Video frame processing with MobileNetV3 for real-time surveillance. J. Comput. Vis. (2024)
35. Kim, S., Park, J.: Integrating MobileNetV3 in autonomous vehicle systems: real-time detection and tracking. IEEE Access (2024)
36. Lin, Y., Xu, R.: Power-efficient AI: a case study of MobileNetV3 in embedded systems. J. Embed. Syst. (2024)
37. Sun, K., Zhang, Q.: Explainable AI in mobile devices: unpacking the decisions of MobileNetV3. Expert Syst. Appl. (2024)
38. Smith, J., Liu, X.: Evaluating machine learning models: beyond accuracy. J. Mach. Learn. Res. (2024)
39. Patel, A., Wang, R.: Precision and recall trade-offs in AI systems: a critical analysis. IEEE Trans. Artif. Intell. (2024)
40. Chen, L., Zhang, Y.: Measuring recall in imbalanced datasets: a case study. Int. J. Comput. Vis. (2024)
41. Davis, T., Sun, M.: The role of F1 score in model evaluation: a comparative study. Pattern Recogn. Lett. (2024)
42. Zhao, Q., He, L.: ROC and AUC metrics: a deep dive into their use in AI model assessment. J. Artif. Intell. Res. (2024)
43. Kim, H., Park, J.: Comprehensive performance evaluation of machine learning models in real-world applications. Expert Syst. Appl. (2024)
44. Zhang, Y., Liu, P.: Leveraging flutter for AI-powered mobile applications: a framework overview. IEEE Trans. Mob. Comput. (2024)
45. Kim, H., Park, J.: Integrating TensorFlow lite with flutter for offline AI applications. J. Artif. Intell. Res. (2024)
46. Wang, T., Zhao, F.: Cloud-based AI in flutter: applications and performance evaluation. IEEE Access (2024)
47. Li, Q., Chen, L.: AI-enhanced user experiences in mobile health applications using flutter. J. Biomed. Inf. (2024)
48. Patel, A., Sun, M.: Real-time decision making in smart systems with AI-powered flutter apps. Expert Syst. Appl. (2024)
49. Davis, T., Zhang, K.: Cross-platform development of AI-driven mobile applications using flutter. Pattern Recogn. Lett. (2024)

Examining Personalized Explainable Recommendations that Support College Students on Stress Management

Mamatha Putta and Jomara Sandbulte[✉]

University of Minnesota Duluth, Duluth, MN, USA
{putta012,jsandbul}@d.umn.edu

Abstract. College students face many challenges, including life transitions and academic and social stressors, which can impact their overall well-being. Digital mental health (DMH) tools can assist in managing these stressors through self-tracking approaches that collect personal data and provide insights into health status. However, to effectively help individuals to manage stress, it is crucial to offer direct guidance on actionable steps for change. To explore this domain, we developed a system with an automated recommendation feature as a technology probe to investigate how personalized health recommendations can support college students in stress management. We conducted a user study with 20 college students to learn from their experiences. Our analysis reveals participants' insights on the effectiveness of recommendations in motivating self-care and the benefits of using personalized recommendations to guide individual actions. Based on our findings, we discuss strategies and design implications to further support college students in managing stress.

Keywords: College Students · Stress Management · Personalized Recommendations · Explanation · Technology Probe · Wearable · User Study

1 Introduction

Recent reports have shown that mental health issues are growing both in severity and prevalence among emerging adults in the U.S [2]. Although people of all ages can be affected by poor mental health, these concerns are particularly higher among college students. A national survey in the USA revealed that 36% of freshmen students in college feel overwhelmed and stressed and may develop severe chronic levels of distress [28,50]. In addition, college students have reported that their mental health was negatively impacted by the COVID-19 pandemic [41,47,57]. While the pandemic heightened existing stressors for students, it also introduced new concerns such as social isolation [41,47]. Prior studies have reported college students' stressors including college life and continuous deadlines, staying away from home, and neglecting self care [26]. This has led to a number of research explorations on how to leverage existing tools to understand students' conditions [32,56], improve students' access to mental health resources [59], and how to timely alleviate college students' mental health state [60].

Digital mental health (DMH) interventions have been explored to support students' well-being [31,40,54]. For instance, the MindNavigator workshop featured a series of events aimed at understanding stress and developing personalized strategies to manage it, encouraging self-experimentation [35]. Additionally, Kazi and Sandbulte [25] proposed a mobile app that focuses on students' social interactions and self-reported stress levels and preferred activities to offer tailored recommendations. Moreover, Yoo and De Choudhury [60] introduced a dashboard design intended to help understand students' mental health by providing timely support. Digital interventions are increasingly important for stress management as students integrate technology-supported mental health strategies into their daily routines [29,31]. Kruzan et al. [29] found that while users value self-tracking technologies for managing mental health symptoms, they often abandon these tools because they lack actionable strategies or insights. To address this gap, self-tracking tools need to provide not only data-driven feedback but also direct *guidance* and *prompts for action* [4,8].

This study seeks to fill this gap by investigating how personalized recommendations can effectively prompt individuals to take action in their self-care. We thus developed *FreeMind: Health Tracker (HT)* – a technology probe designed to explore how personalized health recommendations can aid college students in managing stress. Inspired by prior works [12,26,30], the FreeMind: HT application employs an expert system to suggest effective behavioral strategies in stress management [19,21,51]. To guide this study, we propose the following research questions:

RQ.1: *"How might an explainable recommendation system influence people's decision to take action in the context of stress management ?"*
RQ.2: *"What pros and cons arguments do people have on receiving personalized explainable recommendations for stress management ?"*

To address our research questions, we conducted a user study with 20 college students to examine their perceptions of the explainable recommendations and to determine if these recommendations would effectively prompt them to action towards stress management. Participants interacted with two versions of the *FreeMind:HT* probe: one that included sensor data and one that did not. Following the study, participants compared the two versions in terms of user experience, satisfaction, and the effectiveness of explainable recommendations to promote well-being.

Overall, participants gave positive feedback about the FreeMind: HT recommendations. The sensor-integrated version was particularly highlighted, as its recommendations, based on wearable data, significantly motivated participants to engage in self-care practices. Additionally, our results include examples of participants taking action after receiving recommendations from the intervention. Participants also suggested improving the timing and context of these recommendations to enhance their relevance and effectiveness.

In sum, this study advances the fields of health informatics, wearable technology in healthcare, and technology design by examining the impact of explainable recommendations on individuals' personal health. It also provides insights into effectively supporting college students in managing stress. Additionally, we offer recommendations for enhancing the role of wearable devices in addressing healthcare challenges based on user experiences.

2 Related Work

To investigate individuals' perceptions of personalized recommendations in health technologies, this study builds on previous research on recommendation explainability, health interventions with intelligent computing, and managing stress during college years.

2.1 College Students and Stress Management

Every individual deals with stress at various stages of life. However, college students are a critical group since they are in the stage of life where mental health issues are most probable to occur [26,35]. For many students, the stress of being separated from their family, staying in completely new place, and academic pressure can exacerbate their mental condition [43,56]. In addition, college students have reported that their mental health was negatively impacted by the COVID-19 pandemic [41,47,57].

This critical situation has led to a number of explorations as to how the field of Human-Computer Interaction (HCI) can leverage existing platforms to understand students' conditions [32,44], improve access to mental health resources [59], and provide support for college students' mental health [27,60]. In addition, there is an increased interest in the potential for a more holistic technology design to support important mental well-being factors to increase the effectiveness of mental health interventions [53,54]. Thus, we follow recent advances in this research scope to examine digital interventions to support college students' in stress management.

2.2 Technological Solutions to Support College Students' Well-Being

Mental well-being has various definitions and is a concept that has been studied in multiple fields [53,54]. One characteristic that spans multiple conceptualizations is that mental well-being is fundamental to one's general health and quality of life, and enables us to build resilience against everyday stresses [53,54]. Within HCI, studies have explored mental well-being in different contexts and populations, including college students [12,40,44]. For example, Koustuv and De Choudhury used social media data to assess the mental well-being of college students [44]. And Lattie et al., [32] investigation presented considerations for designing digital mental health tools to support college students mental health.

Prior works have also used passively sensed data from smartphones and wearables and machine learning (ML) techniques to make inferences about an individual's mental status. For example, BeWell [30] is a smartphone well-being app, which monitors user behavior along three health dimensions, namely sleep, physical activity, and social interaction. Another example is the Motivate application that provides personalized and contextualized advice on physical activities [37]. In addition, Morshed et al., [40] study used sensing data from mobile and wearable devices to predict user's mood instabilities.

Particularly for college student's mental health, Egilmez et al. [12], study investigated how a wristwatch could be used to detect stress levels of college students. Wang et al., [56] conducted a long-term study to track depression dynamics in college students using mobile phone and wearable sensing. Finally, the Mindscope is an algorithm-assisted stress management system to support user-driven self-insight [26]. These prior studies effectively demonstrate how sensor data can predict behaviors [30,40] and ML techniques can be applied to identify patterns to provide tailored support [26,37].

While recent technological advances have improved healthcare delivery, still it is important to consider existing concerns about bias in the development of mobile health technologies. For example, Velichkovska et al., [55] study reported cases of different forms of bias in medical technology design and its impact on quality of care provided. And Abràmoff et al., [1] proposed a framework to educate stakeholders on how potential AI/ML bias may impact healthcare outcomes.

Building on design strategies from previous works and recent advances, we developed a passive sensing system to extract information on users' behavior and generate personalized recommendations to support their well-being. Our recommendation format is inspired by explanation styles found in the literature [4,13,46]. Also, the explanations contain behavioral suggestions on how one can manage stress to inform individual action towards mental well-being [4,13].

2.3 Health Interventions with Intelligent Computing

Since smartphones and wearable devices contain onboard sensors that track activity (e.g., movement) and physiological functions (e.g., heart rate), prior studies have utilize passive sensing data and ML methods to study and make inferences about an individual's health in a more personalized manner [7,8,16,26,39,40]. For example, the GlucoGoalie application helps individuals with chronic conditions like type 2 diabetes (T2D) to set goals for improving their diet and work towards achieving these goals [16]. The study's findings showed that receiving goal suggestions augmented participants' self-discovery and the experience of following goals demonstrated the importance of feedback and context [16]. Additionally, Coppens etal., [7] conducted a randomized controlled trial study to investigate motivation of sedentary people when receiving personalized recommendations to move more. The study's findings suggested that the personalized recommendations increased people's motivation to break sedentary behavior [7].

In the mental health context, some studies have used smartphone sensor data to detect the presence and severity of mental health disorders, including depression [56]. One example is the EmotiCal system which uses past mood data to model and visualize future user moods with the goal of encouraging participants to adopt remedial new behaviors to regulate negative moods before they occur [22]. Another example is the StressSense mobile application with a sensing system that uses the phone's built-in microphone to capture human speech during social interactions to infer a user's level of perceived stressed by analyzing para-linguistic information, such as pitch and speaking rate [38]. The aforementioned studies suggest that personal mental-health sensing platforms with sufficient accuracy can enhance mental health care by identifying individuals in need of treatment, particularly those whose conditions involve a loss of motivation, stigmatization, and a sense of hopelessness, which can interfere with seeking help [39, 56].

While these platforms increase user awareness of their health through data-driven information, they are less effective in changing unhealthy habits. This is because they focus on symptom monitoring rather than providing actionable strategies or insights to better support mental health, which can ultimately make individuals feel worse and lead them to abandon smart devices [14, 29, 33]. To motivate healthy habits, systems should guide users on actions to change or mitigate unwanted outcomes [17, 31]. Therefore, it is crucial to provide direct guidance that effectively informs and motivates individual action toward self-care, in addition to offering data-driven feedback such as trends and patterns [4, 16, 29, 37]. Without such strategies, mental-health sensing platforms will continue to fall short in prompting positive changes for mental well-being [17, 29, 31, 40].

2.4 Recommendation Explainability

Prior works have reported that as intelligent computing systems increasingly mediate consequential decision-making, their explainability is critical for end-users to take informed and accountable actions [13, 46]. Additionally, explanations can influence the acceptability of personalized recommendations [42]. However, research on explainable recommendations has shown that explanations are not "one-size-fits-all"; their form and function depend on the context, user personalization, and adaptive capability [10, 11, 36, 42].

For example, the Mindscope application provides explainable recommendations to elucidate how stress levels are computed based on the user's daily activities captured by a smartphone [26]. The study suggests that systems could adjust the levels of explainability according to the amount of data collected and the accuracy of the model to avoid negatively affecting the user experience [26]. Another example is the Kaya application [15], which investigates how current AI descriptions influence individuals' attitudes towards algorithmic recommendations in fertility self-tracking. The study results showed that, despite a general preference for tools with descriptive AI, users reported that they would not blindly trust the algorithmic process [15].

Based on these prior findings [11,13,26,46], our system generates automated recommendations based on users' data. These recommendations include explanations to provide reasons for the predictions, aiming to increase recommendation acceptance and prompt informed actions [10,42,46]. The explanations incorporate stress relief strategies found in the literature to be effective in managing stress [21,51].

3 System Design

Technology probes are a method often used to understand individual's needs in a real-world setting and inspire people to imagine the use of the new technology [9,23,24]. We developed a technology probe called *FreeMind: Health Tracker (HT)* which provides personalized recommendations to encourage users to take action on self-care. FreeMind:HT was developed using Flutter[1] Flutter is an open source framework created by Google and it is used to develop cross-platform applications for Android, iOS, etc. from a single code base. We also used Django framework[2] which is an open-source, Python-based web framework to build the application back-end. Finally, we used Garmin Smartwatch[3] which is a commercial available device to collect the user's daily activity levels including stress and sleep levels. The FreeMind:HT application had two versions:

- **Base Version**: Application *without* the sensor model.
- **Sensor-based Version**: Application *with* the sensor model.

The Base Version application includes a homepage where users can post and view pictures of their daily activities (see Fig. 1 - A). To generate the recommendation, users are prompted to answer a survey to report their preferences on various activities and well-being assessment. The Base Version application generates an automated recommendation based on users' survey response (see Fig. 1 - B). Inspired by prior works [19,32], the application presents information on existing health services from our local institution within the app to facilitate people help-seeking behaviors (see Fig. 1 - C).

The FreeMind:HT Sensor-Based Version *includes all design features* from the Base Version, extending it by including the sensing data to generate the recommendations.

3.1 Application Model

The proposed system is composed by two main parts: a sensor module and a recommendation module. The sensor module uses data from a Garmin device.

---

[1] Flutter: https://flutter.dev/.
[2] Django: https://www.djangoproject.com/.
[3] Garmin: https://www.garmin.com/en-US/.

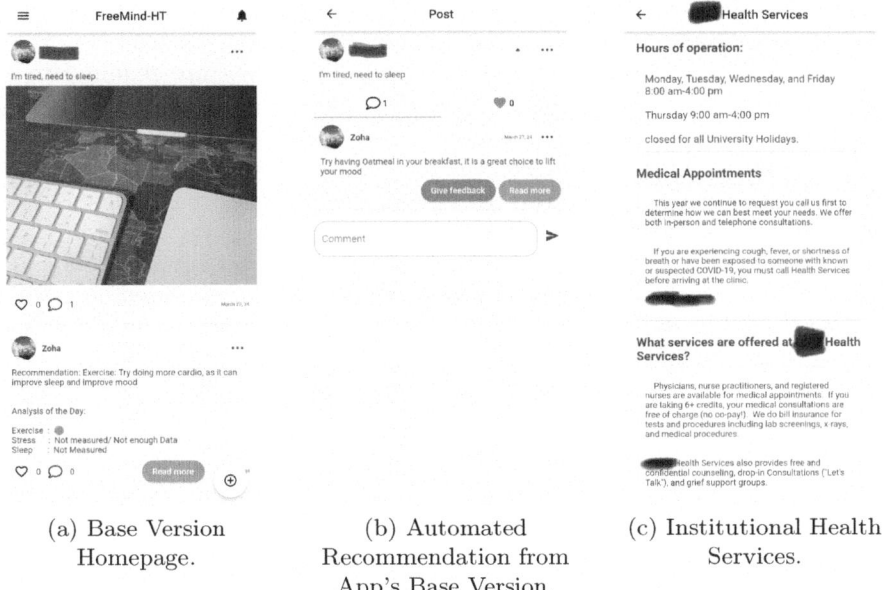

(a) Base Version Homepage. (b) Automated Recommendation from App's Base Version. (c) Institutional Health Services.

Fig. 1. FreeMind:HT Base Version Overview. a) Users can post and view pictures of their daily activities; b) the application generates an automated recommendation based on users' survey response; c) the application includes information on existing health services from our local institution.

We selected Garmin after reviewing consumer smartwatches in terms of their accuracy, ease-of-use, battery life, and the presence of features designed for the sensing data collection. Garmin provides a developer portal with access to the user activity data and sleep data.

Based on prior works [39,61], we decided to leverage existing algorithms and techniques to build our application' recommendation module instead of improving the accuracy of recommender systems or technical precision. The recommendation module uses a collaborative filtering algorithm to recommend activities [61]. This algorithm finds the most similar user to a particular user. Based on the most similar users, the model estimates the ratings for each activity in the activity pool [52,61]. We leveraged data from prior works to define our activity pool and labels for the activities [8,25,45]. Sample activities are: Spend time in nature, Going to the Gym, Drinking water, Eating fruit and vegetables.

Following others strategies [25,26], we used user's survey data to feed the recommendation module to address the cold start issue. We also added some constrains within the system to avoid recommending the same activity multiple times in a row. Finally, our recommendation system is not continuously learning about the user.

The proposed recommender system uses two data entries: a) the user's survey data and b) sensor data to extract meaningful information on users' behavior to make personalized recommendations. The user's survey collects the user's preferences on various activities and self-report well-being assessment [48]. When the user creates an account within the application, they are required to fill out this survey to feed the model. After that, the user can start wearing the smartwatch together with the application which allows the system to track the user' vitals and activity level. Then, the application combines both data entries (i.e., survey data along with the data generated by the wearable sensor) to analyze the user activity level throughout the day.

Finally, the system generates a recommendation and posts it at the application homepage. The recommendation contains an *explanation* based on descriptive styles found in the literature [13,26,46]. The explanation's content consists of a suggestion on how to manage stress to inform individual action towards well-being [4,26].

Sensor Module. To analyze the user's daily activity level, the system collects data from a commercially available smartwatch, namely Garmin device. The smartwatch's sensor collects user data from an extensive array of data attributes. For this study, we extracted the following key attributes: calories, steps, stress analysis and sleep duration.

After proper user authentication, the Garmin developer portal provides access to user's daily activity data and sleep data. The daily activity data contains details about the user's caloric activity, steps count, stress analysis of the user's day (i.e., 'stressful', 'unknown', 'balanced', 'calm', 'balanced_awake', 'default'). And the sleep data has the sleep analysis such as total hours of sleep and sleep qualifiers (i.e., 'poor', 'fair', 'good', 'excellent'). Table 1 presents the sleep and daily activity data to infer the user's daily activity.

Recommendation System. After collecting data from the smartwatch, the model analyses the user's daily activity level based on four data-points: sleep, calories, steps, stress level. These data points can be attributed to the rest that the user got, the amount of exercise the user indulged in, and the user's daily stress level. The model analyses the activity data to generate prioritization scores for the activities. These scores are generated to make a 10% or 30% increase in the activity that is not satisfactorily performed on a day or to make a decrease of 20% in the activity that is not satisfactorily performed on a day (see Table 1 and the example provided in Sect. 3.1).

We defined these percentages for increase/decrease after evaluating the model with three rounds of rigorous testing. We tested three different increase/decrease percentage values, intending to find a optimal prioritization percentage for the model. Each round of the testing included all possible combinations of a daily activity which resulted in 36 combinations (3*3*4=36) of daily activity levels (see Table 1).

Our activity group contains three items: sleep, stress, and exercise. A score ranging from 0 to 2 is generated to each item of the activity group based on the analysis of the model. These scores are then passed on to the recommendation

Table 1. Range of values for each of the activities

Exercise ([18, 20, 51])	• Sedentary day: 0–300 calories & 0–5000 steps • Active day: 300–500 calories & 5000–10000 steps • Very Active day: greater than 500 cal & greater than 10000 steps
Sleep ([21, 49])	• Not enough sleep: less than 7 h • Enough sleep: 7–9 hours • Restful: greater than 9 h
Stress (from Garmin)	• Stressful • Balanced • Calm • unknown: Stress not measured by the app or not enough data is available for the day to provide stress analysis

model. The recommendation system then takes into account the priority score generated by the sensor model and the scores generated by collaborative filtering algorithm to multiply them and then, generate the final recommendation list. Thus, the activities are prioritized according to the user's preference and the sensor activity data. The recommendation with a highest score is considered the final recommendation that the user will receive as a post on the home screen of the app (see Fig. 2).

How the System Generates the Recommendations: Here is an example to explain the system process in detail: Imagine the following scenario where a user has burned less than 300 cal, has taken less than 5000 steps, has slept well (i.e., sleep duration is 8 h), and the stress analysis is Calm. In this scenario, based on the analysis of our model, the scores for each activity group would be as follows:

– Exercise Score: 1.3;
– Food Score: 1;
– Sleep Score: 1;
– Stress Score: 0.8.

These scores are used to prioritize the recommendations. Now, if the exercise recommendation has a score of 4, then that recommendation is prioritized with a multiplicity of 1.3 and the final score for that exercise recommendation would be 5.2. Once all the recommendations are multiplied with their group multiplicity, they will then be sorted to recommend an activity with the highest score. To make sure that the same recommendation is not being recommended repeatedly, we defined a constraint within the system to not send a recommendation from the last 10 received.

3.2 Recommendation Explainability Style

The FreeMind:HT system includes an automated recommendation with an explanation that contains a behavioral strategy to relief stress and encourage students' well-being [4,13]. Some of those relievers are: engaging in physical activities to help manage stress, eating healthy and nutritious food, and behaviors to improve sleep quality [43,51,58]. Users receive a recommendation on the application home page of their account with the suggested activity based on their personal data collected (see Fig. 2 - A).

The system's recommendation template was inspired in [25,36] and consists of three parts: a) the activity recommendation itself, b) the reasoning of the system behind the generating that activity as a recommendation, and c) the analysis of the day. The recommendation template is listed below:

"Recommendation: [activity]: [Activity suggestion] [Analysis of the Day]".

Below, we show an example of an automated recommendation. In the example provided, the red marker associated with exercise represents that the user has not exercised enough during that day and the green marker associated with sleep indicates that the user had sufficient duration of sleep (refer Table 1).

Recommendation: Exercise: "Try going to the Gym, it improves physical well-being and mood."
Analysis of the Day:
Exercise:
Stress: Not measured/Not enough data
Sleep: Analysis: GOOD

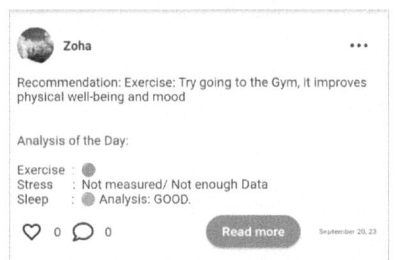
(a) Example of a recommendation with the analysis of the day.

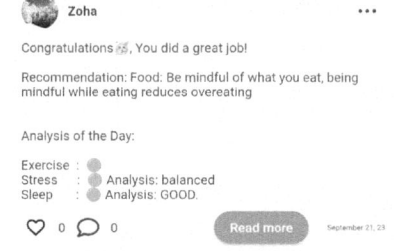
(b) Example of a recommendation with the positive reinforcement.

Fig. 2. Examples of the Recommendation Explanations

Finally, when the user manages a day well, the analysis of the day is all good (i.e., the markers are all green). Then, our system provides a positive comment to encourage the users as suggested in the literature [25,29]. For example, when a user had burned calories greater than or equal to 300 while reaching the minimum sleep goal of seven hours and also maintaining the stress within the balanced/calm state, then the user will receive a message congratulating them for the well performed day as shown in Fig. 2 - B. Users can read more about the activity' benefits and resources available within the institution by clicking at the "Read More" button.

4 Methods

Given our interest in understanding the students' perceptions on personalized recommendations and its benefits to help managing stress, we conducted a two-day long user study to observe participants' practices on using the proposed technology probe in their natural settings and test the application under realistic conditions [34]. We decided the study's duration based on prior short-term deployment studies and not to be a significant barrier for recruitment [25,45].

4.1 Study Design and Recruitment

This research was approved by the Institutional Review Board (IRB) before beginning any research activity. We recruited participants from our local institution by posting fliers around the university (e.g., library, bulletin boards) and through word of mouth. We defined as inclusion criteria: a) Individuals 18+ years old and b) Individuals enrolled as a student in our local institution. Recruitment continued until data saturation was reached, defined as the point at which no new themes emerged during the data analysis.

Participants interacted with the system for two-days long and were awarded with $30 compensation at the end of the study. Each study session was conducted in-person and the interview session lasted around one hour. Each participant sequentially interacted with two versions of the application: with and without the sensor model, as presented below in details:

- **Base Version**: Application interaction *without* the sensor model for a full-day. And, a follow-up survey to log user experience with the app.
- **Sensor-based Version**: Application interaction *with* the sensor model for a full-day. And, a follow-up survey to log user experience with the app.

The order of the interaction was randomized. We defined as the independent variables of the study: having and not having the sensor data from the wearable. And as dependent variable, we considered the user experience and satisfaction based on the following metrics:

- How relevant were the recommendations made by each model?
- Which recommendation model motivated users more to take action towards self-care?
- How satisfied were the users with the application?

After using both the versions for a full-day (from 9–10 am to 5–6 pm), we conducted in-person interview session with each participant where they could share more about their experience with the application.

4.2 Participants Overview

A total of 20 people participated in our study. 9 participants were male, 11 were female participants. 10 participants were graduate students and 10 were undergraduate students. 9 of the participants self-identified as Asian and 9 self-identified as White and the other 2 identified themselves into multiple races. The age range was 19–36 years old ($M = 25.5$, $SD = 5.2$). Finally, all participants reported experience using mobile phones as experts.

In terms of using the local institution health services resources, 75.0% (15 out of 20) participants said to not have used any services and 25.0% (5 out of 20) participants said to have used some services such as counseling services and grief support group.

In terms of perceived stress level, 60% (12 out of 20) participants reported experiencing stress and nervousness about half or more than half of the time. For all participants, the perceived stress level was $M = 3.15$, $SD = 1.14$ (on a scale of 5).

4.3 Data Collection

We followed the described procedure for this study data collection. First, we offered introductory remarks which included a concise overview of the study, and sought verbal consent from participants. Upon receiving their consent, we demonstrated the application and showed how to use the wearable device through both screenshots and hands-on examples on a mobile device. Subsequently, participants were given the opportunity to personally explore the application.

We loaned the mobile and wearable devices for the duration of the study. Over a span of two days, each participant was assigned to use the two different versions of the application, one each day. Initially, half of the participants, totaling 10 individuals, engaged with the Base Version on the first day and transitioned to Sensor-based Version on the subsequent day. The remaining 10 participants followed a reverse sequence, starting with Sensor-based Version and then switching to Base Version.

Assigned tasks varied depending on the version in use. For the Base Version, participants were required to make photo posts within the application at least three times (i.e., morning, afternoon, and evening) during the study day when convenient. For the Sensor-based Version, participants needed to synchronize data collected by their Garmin sensor with the Garmin mobile application three times a day (at least), following a predetermined morning, afternoon, and evening schedule. We asked participants their preferred time to sync the devices. Thus, each participant received at least six recommendations throughout the study (i.e., three recommendations from each version).

After spending a day with the application, participants were required to complete a Qualtrics survey to share their experience with that particular version. Some sample questions are: *"Did you feel more motivated to stay healthy while using the app?"*; *"On a scale of 0 to 10, how satisfied were you with this model of the recommendation app you used?"* This process was repeated for the other version on the following day, with an additional survey completed at the end of the second day to gather comparative feedback on both versions.

Concluding the study, we conducted one-on-one interviews with participants to collect their feedback on both versions. Some sample questions from the interview are: *"Tell us your thoughts about the recommendation. How useful was it to inspire you to take action for your well-being ?"*; *"How relevant was the recommendation to your day? Give us an example."* and *"How did the explanation provided by the app help you in understanding the stress pattern? and how did it affect your motivation to take action?"* This step was crucial in understanding their overall user experience and in comparing the two versions directly.

4.4 Data Analysis

For this study, we want to understand how personalized recommendations may affect people's decision to take action for self-care. We collected the following data during this study: a) observations notes from participants' interactions within the application; b) participants' responses to the surveys; c) participants' comments about the system from an interview session.

We employed thematic analysis as proposed in [6]. The interview data was transcribed by a third-party service called Parrot AI[4] Each research team member independently reviewed the same transcripts, notes from the data collection, and looked deeper into them for interesting findings. The research team coded the data and met regularly to discuss it and generate an initial codebook. Then, the codebook was iteratively revised to better encompass the data until the findings were pieced together into themes. Finally, we applied peer-debriefing, agreed upon a set of code, and group them together into relevant themes.

The themes include data related to the user's impressions on the application design, preferences on the recommendations and its effectiveness to motivate action towards self- care, recommendations impact on users' decision-making, and benefits for stress management.

5 Results

In this section, we summarize the major themes and factors under the themes derived from our qualitative analysis. Our analysis considered participants' experience with the application and sought to answer the study's research questions. We identify participants by a P followed by a number.

5.1 Application Feedback

We gathered participants' impressions of the *FreeMind:HT* design and functions. While the study was not specifically focused on usability, this feedback is still valuable for understanding the overall user experience.

During the interviews, participants commented on the recommendations visual representation, specifically the use of green and red markers for daily

---

[4] Parrot AI: https://parrot.ai/.

analysis, to be motivating and helpful in understanding their day. The daily report feature was noted for its ease readability and utility in monitoring health status (P9). Participant 10 said: *"I liked the visual of the dots. I really liked being able to see ...it's kind of checking the box on a list... kind of a satisfying little check mark."* (P10) This comment suggests that the application's design successfully communicated key information at a glance.

In terms of areas of improvement, participants presented helpful suggestions to enhance the system design such as expand the color scale for daily analysis to provide a better understanding of the data and more accurately represent the degree of completion of the task (P9). Participants suggested that the system could incorporate 'fun' small activities such as jokes, cat videos, and puzzles to aid stress management (P16,P18). For example, participant P18 said: *"Recommendations like watching funny videos or getting brief clips of content I enjoy, like cat videos, personalized based on my preferences, would significantly aid stress management."* (P18) The recommendations could also include quick, fun activities such as relaxation techniques, reminders to connect with family, or deep breathing exercises for immediate stress relief (P1, P5, P12, P18, P20).

This is a particularly interesting feedback since students have a busy schedule and time consuming tasks may not always be achievable. As participant 12 explained that their stress comes from daily academic pressure which prevents them to engage in self-care activities: *"... a lot of my stress is school related and so I don't have a lot of time because it's such a strict timeline. So it'd be nice [since] a lot of recommendations are short, quick things to do, like breathing exercises. So it's like, 'oh, just take a minute and do this instead'."* (P12)

Finally, participants suggested that goal-setting and gamification (P8, P10, P13) could enhance the user experience. For example, participant P10 said that setting goals for drinking water could affect their motivation to stay hydrated: *"if your goal was to drink more water, then your watch could say 'hey, how are you doing on that water intake?' And it'd be cool if it was like personalized where you could every time it asked you could add how much water you've drank. So then you can try to reach your goal."* (P10)

5.2 Analysis of the Recommendations Effectiveness to Motivate Self-care

During our interviews, we encouraged participants to share pros and cons arguments on receiving the recommendations (RQ.2) We also analyzed the recommendations affect on participants' motivation to take action towards self-care (RQ.1). When comparing the FreeMind:HT two versions, it was clear that integrating the wearable sensor module greatly improved the relevance and applicability of health recommendations, leading to increased motivation for participants to engage in self-care practices. Figure 3 shows participants responses to the end of the experiment survey.

When reflecting on their experience with the Base Version, participants mentioned its value for offering advice that feels personally relevant, especially in terms of users' emotional well-being and serving as a friend for guidance (P14,

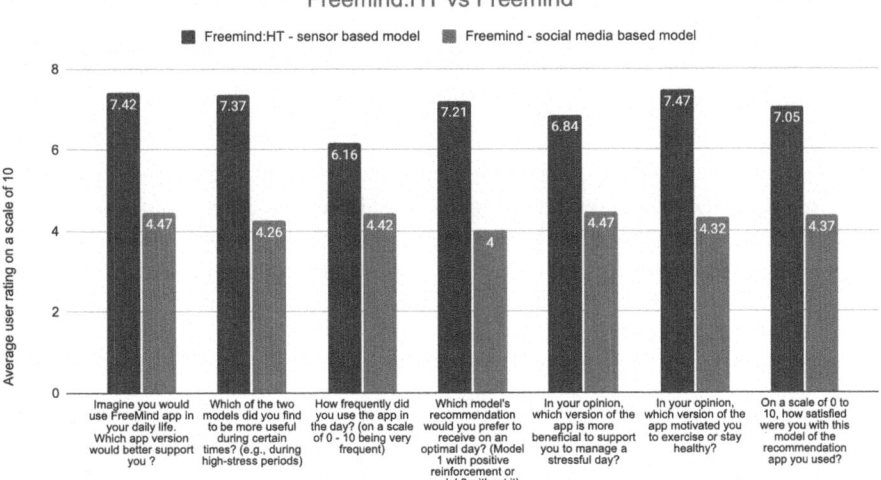

Fig. 3. Survey data comparing the application versions. Blue columns represent the Sensor-based Version. Red columns represent the Base Version. (Color figure online)

P17). For example, participant 17 said that the system provided a friendly recommendation: *"...when I posted about my stress, it recommend a best recommendation for control my stress. I thought I have a friend that she is gonna help me or give me some good advice for controlling my stress."* (P17). This insight highlights the unique advantage of the non-sensor model in providing empathetic and personalized advice. However, integrating sensors could potentially offer a more comprehensive and precise approach to healthcare by incorporating real-time physical health data.

Additionally, our analysis shows that the Sensor-based Version was preferred since it provided recommendations that closely aligned with the users' physical states and immediate health needs. Specifically, 35% (7 out of 20) of participants reported that the sensor integration enhanced their understanding of their health data, allowing the model to deliver advice that was both relevant and actionable during crucial moments. For instance, participant 19 shared their experience with the Sensor-based Version: *"...the app recommendations about what I got after or while I was asleep that was helpful because it said 'try getting better sleep, sleep affects human bodies in different ways'. I didn't get much sleep. And then I got one it was 'try drinking more water'. The time that I was using this, I was in the lab. It felt like It knew what I was doing."* (P19)

Still, some participants (4 out of 20) mentioned that the Sensor-based Version's recommendations could benefit from improved contextual timing. For example, participant P16 explained that they received a recommendation about socializing that was not relevant to their current context: *"... one of the recommendation came before I went to class and it said, 'to try socializing', but I was about to go to a class where I can't really do that. So that was like, it would have been a great suggestion if I had more free time afterwards. Some of the suggestions just didn't really work for what I was about to do." (P16)*

As follows, we present details into the various ways the sensor-integrated model influenced our participants, including increased motivation and feelings of support, and making healthier lifestyle choices after receiving recommendations.

Recommendation Impact on User's Motivation. Participants mentioned to have experienced a notable boost in motivation due to the sensor module's approach to positive reinforcement. Congratulatory messages for achievements seemed to serve as a efficient tool for encouragement since this approach not only acknowledges their achievements but also encourages them to maintain and build upon their healthy habits. For example, participant 10 mentioned his thoughts on the positive reinforcement messages: *"I liked that. It, after I worked out, it told me. 'Congratulations' which was cool. I thought that was cute." (P10).* In addition, the use of visual cues, such as red and green markers, served as an immediate and intuitive form of feedback *"I say yeah, especially because of sleep because it's red and I usually like towards the end of the day, see myself getting more drowsy and whatnot. So that does show the you know, like a correlation." (P15)*, further reinforcing positive behavior and making the tracking progress engaging and rewarding.

The sensor-model's ability to identify stress and offer supportive recommendations was also well-received for its role in promoting optimism and showcasing effective stress management strategies (P8, P13, P18), for instance participant P18 said that receiving a supportive recommendation was helpful during a difficult day: *"'Be Optimistic', okay. That was very helpful for me because it suggested positivity when I was feeling down during a long weekend at home." (P18).* Our participants explained that this approach not only supports their stress management but also encourages them to undertake healthful activities.

Recommendation Impact on User's Decision-Making. Since our system was designed to provide direct guidance for promoting a healthier lifestyle, recommendations to engage in physical activities like walking and hiking, as well as eating more fruits and vegetables, proved particularly effective. 35% (7 out of 20) of the participants reported increased engagement in these activities, which they might not have pursued otherwise. For example, participant 13 mentioned that they <u>received and followed</u> a suggestion from the system: *"Well, [I follow] lots of stuff that go out in nature. So I tried going on hiking trails and stuff. So just part of nature." (P13)* Similarly, participant 18 mentioned <u>taking action</u> by making some food after receiving a recommendation: *"Yeah, I actually got food. I went, because I realized I hadn't eaten all day. And then this app is saying that, then I should probably do it. So I went and made a sandwich." (P18)*

In addition, participants suggested that the study intervention helped them on decision-making towards their health. For example, participant 16 explained that during a stressful day, it is hard to decide how to cope: *"I think I were feeling like, 'oh, I feel a little bit stressful or worried' and I just couldn't decide* what to do because sometimes I get in those moods where I don't know if I want to sit here and relax or if I wanna go do something just like to sink it.

Participant 16 further explained that the guidance provided by the system served as a self-care reminder since it offered a practical strategy that benefits their health: "... sometimes I skip meals and just have snacks and having it remind me to have a healthy meal was definitely helpful and I would be more likely to take the initiative to make a healthy meal." (P16)

5.3 Benefits of Personalized Recommendations for Stress Management

In our study, participants reflected on their experiences receiving personalized recommendations to manage stress based on our study metrics (RQ.2).

20% (4 out of 20) of the participants found the Base Version to be more effective since its recommendations were more related to the participant's post: "The 'without sensor module' seemed more responsive and relevant to my posts and feelings." (P17). Also, participants appreciated the varied suggestions based on their manual entries "The 'without sensor module' gave me more varied suggestions, which I found helpful." (P16), which provided a different but still effective form of stress management support.

80% (16 out of 20) of the participants reported a preference for the system "with the sensor module" to support stress management. For example, participant P10 said the sensor data helped to track health status: "I feel like I wasn't too stressed to begin with, but the 'with sensor module' probably helped maintain that even on similar days."(P10) The Sensor-based version aided participants in being more proactive about their health behaviors to cope with stress. For example, participant P20 mentioned how the system encouraged self-care: "It's better. I'm not a person who tracks my walking and things like that, but if it reminds me about that [tracking], it is better to eat something, some food, it's better for me." (P20).

Participants appreciated the visual elements of the system with a sensor module (i.e., green and red dots) and reported its influence on their motivation to manage their stress: "I like the visualization-it motivated me to turn the red mark to green." (P8). The ability to 'see the stress levels' helped participants to actively think on how to address it: "Seeing the visualized indicators helped me think about reducing my stress actively." (P9). And empower them on finding strategies to cope with stress: "It was motivating to see that there are ways to effectively handle stress." (P13) Similar feedback was also echoed by others (P6, P16, P17, P18, P19), highlighting the effect of the recommendations during the experiment.

However, our participants mentioned that the provided guidance can improve its credibility by including research articles to make the advice not only relevant but also reliable. For example, participant P10 said: "If It had like, links to new research or things would spike your interest versus I already know that I should probably be eating better. But if it's like a new research study that shows this, this and this, I would definitely want to know more about all that." (P10)

Finally, 30% (6 out of 20) of participants suggested that the system should offer a broader range of recommendations, including mental health topics, socialization strategies, and relaxation techniques. By providing more diverse and tailored suggestions, the system could better support participants in taking action, whether through exercise, dietary changes, or other healthful practices.

5.4 Feedback on the Recommendations Explanation

We also collected data on participants' impressions on the recommendation explainability. The application's ability to communicate the reasons behind certain recommendations by explaining *why* an activity might help to reduce stress was highlighted as particularly beneficial. For example, participant P4 said: *"Being told by the app that my stress levels are unusually high helps me recognize that it's not normal, which makes the recommendations to address it more credible and urgent." (P4)*. According to our participants, the recommendation explanations were important to support stress management for two main reasons.

First, by showing the poorly performed activities, participants became more aware of how those activities may affect their day. As an example, participant P15 said: *"...because well, for me, when the exercise was red, I was getting more like exercise related recommendations. And also because the sleep is red, I'm getting more of those and those two do improve your stress and like help with sleeping. So yeah, I do see that correlation." (P15)*. Similarly, participant P10 emphasized the importance of understanding the potential factors behind a bad day: *"...because I'd say if my sleep is red and my exercise is red and I'm having a bad day, then I could be like 'this is why I'm probably having a bad day', which is important to be able to figure out." (P10)*

Second, the increased awareness on health status based on sensing data prompted participants to making positive changes. For example, participant P19 explained that during the intervention the system showed that his sleep and exercise levels were low which they associated with having a bad day: *"I think it was helpful because sleep didn't get much. Exercise I didn't get much that day, and it is very true to its results."* After that realization, participant P19 said the increased awareness prompted them to plan self-care activities and motivate them to pursue them: *"... it helped me think about how many hours are in a day and divide the day. Like obviously the night you're gonna sleep for at least eight hours and then for at least one hour of the day, keep that one hour aside for exercising. So like hitting the gym or running, so that one hour is sufficient for the exercise and then the rest of the day is just gonna be what I've usually been doing throughout the day." (P19)*

6 Discussion

This study aimed to explore how personalized recommendations could effectively prompt individuals to focus on their self-care. We developed the *FreeMind:HT* probe as an early version of a technology in a real-world setting to collect data on its use, understand the context of its application, and inspire further development. We then conducted a short-term user study to understand the users' perceptions. Overall, participants responded enthusiastically and had a positive experience while using the *FreeMind:HT* application. According to them, the study experiment provided an opportunity to increase awareness on health needs and think on actionable strategies at critical moments.

Our findings revealed that the application's sensor-based version was particularly effective in providing timely and relevant health recommendations, which were well-received by our participants. Still, participants presented valuable considerations regarding the application base version given its relevance to subjective entries. Although our study scope does not include the evaluation of people's preferences for sensor/non-sensor application, we recommend future work to further examine this line of research.

6.1 Recommendations Influence on People's Decision and Motivation

Our findings indicate that the recommendation suggestions prompted some participants (7 out of 20) to make positive behavioral changes, such as increasing physical activity and adopting healthier eating habits, even during the short-term intervention. Still, a long-term study would be important to observe a comprehensive range of user's behaviors and practices. Nevertheless, our findings provide evidence that can support future design on how real-time monitoring of health dimensions can boost user engagement and how direct guidance can encourage users to take action on well-being.

Additionally, prior interventions that incorporate direct feedback mechanisms are shown to be more engaging and effective in promoting health-related behavioral changes [54]. Our findings extend prior work by using personalized visual cues (i.e., green and red dots) and showing examples on how those cues can serve as motivational features since they provide immediate, easy-to-understand feedback about daily health behaviors [54]. Although the visual feedback with the two-colored markers was well-received, still improving it to include a scale of progress could benefit people with a more nuanced understanding of their daily achievements. Future work could explore design functions that include a gradient color scale that reflects varying levels of health behaviors. Another idea, similar to Koustuv and De Choudhury [44], future systems could use a dashboard that summarizes weekly and monthly progress to give users a clearer long-term perspective of their well-being improvements.

Participants also reported that the application positively influenced their decision-making, encouraging more proactive health and wellness behaviors. For example, participant 18 said how the system's recommendation on healthy eating inspired them to make a sandwich after realizing they had skipped meals. This finding is consistent with Morshed et al. [40], who highlighted how people may use technological interventions to support their decision-making through data-driven insights. Our results illustrate that personalized health recommendations can effectively guide users in making healthier choices by providing relevant suggestions tailored to individual's needs. Inspired by the extensive work on nudges [5], our findings provide additional examples on how well-timed and relevant recommendations may act as effective nudges towards healthier behaviors. We think that a well-designed nudge may significantly influence users' daily behaviors and decision-making processes, thus enhancing the overall effectiveness of the DMH tools [5,32].

6.2 Reflections on Receiving Direct Guidance to Manage Stress

In terms of stress management, prior works have shown the benefits of using personalized recommendations to improve mental well-being, as they cater directly to the user's specific stressors and coping capabilities [3,22,35].

Accordingly, our findings showed that our proposed solution was notably appreciated by participants, who highlighted the tailored nature of the stress management strategies it recommended. Participants presented examples on how the strategies suggested by the system encouraged them to take action. For instance, participant 20 received a recommendation to eat healthy food which inspired them of cooking. Also, participant 19 mentioned how important it was to receive a suggestion to drink water. Thus, our findings contribute with valuable observations of the importance to provide direct guidance that informs individual action on what to do to address unwanted behaviors or outcomes.

However, since our recommendation model is not continuously learning from the user, future iterations could develop algorithm models that allow users to interact more dynamically with the recommendations. For example, the system could allow users to mark tasks as completed. With this direct feedback from the users, the system recommendations would refine its suggestions. We think that this approach could help with the recommendations accuracy and adaptability since it would be based on observed user's long-term behaviors and preferences.

Based on our data, seeing real-time visual feedback on participants' stress levels enabled more immediate and effective interventions, a critical aspect in the fast-paced environments college students often navigate. This finding suggests that interactive and sensor-based health technologies may significantly aid stress management by providing users with actionable and personalized feedback which is in accordance to the literature [7,27,30].

Accordingly, we recommend future technologies to incorporate a more comprehensive array of recommendation types that address various aspects of well-being – including mental, physical, and social health dimensions. For example, future studies could consider integrating individuals' dietary allergies and specific nutritional needs into the food-related recommendations. Additionally, based on our data, the recommendations suggestions could include quick, less time-consuming activities such as watching a short video, playing a brief game, or reading a motivational quote, which could be particularly appealing to people with busy schedules.

Finally, prior studies have shown that users prefer recommendation systems with explanations to understand why they received a prediction [42,46]. While previous works have explored recommendation explainability through speculative design scenarios [13,42], we extend this discussion by providing concrete examples of its effects on participants under realistic conditions. Our data indicates that participants appreciated explanations for why an activity was helpful in reducing stress and felt encouraged to take action towards their well-being, as illustrated by P15's experience. Thus, we argue that providing actionable strategies through explainable recommendations can increase the likelihood of prompting individuals to change and adopt positive behaviors. However, we acknowledge the need for more in-depth exploration into this area of research.

We encourage future studies to build on our proposed system design and assess it through longitudinal studies to better understand its impact on user engagement and explainability acceptance on health recommendations. These studies could help identify patterns over longer periods of time and provide insights into the effectiveness of different types of explanation styles on personal health interventions.

7 Limitations

Our study presents the FreeMind:HT - a technology probe designed to examine how personalized health recommendations can aid college students in managing stress. We are aware of the limitations introduced by our short user study and the preliminary nature of the results since the brief duration of the study may not capture a comprehensive range of user behaviors and responses. Future works are encouraged to conduct long-term interventions to address this issue. Additionally, our research was formative and informed by prior literature with the aim to better understand how a technological intervention may influence people's decision to take action for their well-being, we hope to see future studies focusing on the recommendation system performance and algorithm accuracy.

In addition, we developed different versions of the FreeMind:HT system to investigate how personalized recommendations may influence people's decision to take action towards self-care. Rather than investigating if people prefer a system with or without sensing data collection, we aimed to provide different recommendations based on users' entries and assess their affect on people's perception. Therefore, our results may not extend to preferences towards sensor/non-sensor application. There is opportunity for future studies to pursue this line of research. Besides, similar to Newn et al. [42], we did not intend to evaluate different styles of explanation, but the presence of them. So, we used only one explanation style in our automated recommendation. We are also aware that while asking participants to compare the application versions sequentially to deepen our ability to understand how personalized recommendations influenced perspectives, it also introduced a strong order effect. Still, similar to Figueiredo et al. [15], we were able to answer our research questions effectively because order was randomized and therefore controlled for.

Finally, while we attempted to recruit a larger and diverse sample of students, we are aware that our sample size and group of participants might not be representative of the general population of college students. Also, it is possible that our sample could be biased towards individuals particularly interested in digital mental health tools. Future studies are encouraged to address this limitation. Although our study sample complies with the nature of this research [6], a larger and more diverse sample including participants from broader background is recommended for external validity as it may better represent the general population of college students and a wide spectrum of stress levels. We hope to see future studies addressing this limitation.

8 Conclusion

In this paper, we present findings from a user study aimed at understanding college students' perceptions of personalized recommendations for managing stress. Building on prior works, we developed a recommendation system with explanations to suggest strategies for coping with stress. We conducted a short-term user study with 20 college students to examine how a technological intervention might influence their decisions to take action for their well-being.

Our findings highlight the effectiveness of recommendations in motivating self-care and their impact on students' motivations and decision-making toward a healthier lifestyle. We provide concrete examples of participants taking action toward self-care, demonstrating the benefits of using personalized recommendations for stress management. We argue that providing direct guidance with actionable strategies has significant potential to support individuals in pursuing well-being. Finally, we offer valuable insights for researchers interested in promoting well-being among college students.

Acknowledgments. We would like to thank all the participating students in this study for sharing their experiences. This work was supported by the UMN Early Innovation Fund Program.

References

1. Abràmoff, M.D., et al.: Considerations for addressing bias in artificial intelligence for health equity. NPJ Digital Med. **6**(1), 170 (2023)
2. Abuse, S., (SAMHSA), M.H.S.A.: 2020 national survey on drug use and health - samhsa. https://www.samhsa.gov/data/sites/default/files/reports/rpt35325/NSDUHFFRPDFWHTMLFiles2020/2020NSDUHFFR1PDFW102121.pdf (2020). Accessed 14 Jul 2022
3. Adams, P., et al.: Towards personal stress informatics: Comparing minimally invasive techniques for measuring daily stress in the wild. In: Proceedings of the 8th International Conference on Pervasive Computing Technologies for Healthcare, pp. 72–79. PervasiveHealth '14, ICST (Institute for Computer Sciences, Social-Informatics and Telecommunications Engineering), Brussels, BEL (2014). https://doi.org/10.4108/icst.pervasivehealth.2014.254959
4. Afzal, M., et al.: Personalization of wellness recommendations using contextual interpretation. Expert Syst. Appl. **96**, 506–521 (2018)

5. Bergram, K., Djokovic, M., Bezençon, V., Holzer, A.: The digital landscape of nudging: a systematic literature review of empirical research on digital nudges. In: Proceedings of the 2022 CHI Conference on Human Factors in Computing Systems. CHI '22, Association for Computing Machinery, New York, NY, USA (2022). https://doi.org/10.1145/3491102.3517638
6. Braun, V., Clarke, V.: Successful Qualitative Research: A Practical Guide for Beginners. Sage Publications, UK, London (2013)
7. Coppens, I., Martens, L., De Pessemier, T.: Motivating people to move more with personalized activity and tip recommendations: a randomized controlled trial. In: Companion Proceedings of the 28th International Conference on Intelligent User Interfaces, pp. 123–126. IUI '23 Companion, Association for Computing Machinery, New York, NY, USA (2023). https://doi.org/10.1145/3581754.3584149
8. De Croon, R., Van Houdt, L., Htun, N.N., Štiglic, G., Abeele, V.V., Verbert, K., et al.: Health recommender systems: systematic review. J. Med. Internet Res. **23**(6), e18035 (2021)
9. Derix, E.C., Leong, T.W.: Towards a probe design framework. In: Proceedings of the 31st Australian Conference on Human-Computer-Interaction, pp. 117–127. OZCHI'19, Association for Computing Machinery, New York, NY, USA (2019). https://doi.org/10.1145/3369457.3369467
10. Dhanorkar, S., Wolf, C.T., Qian, K., Xu, A., Popa, L., Li, Y.: Who needs to know what, when?: Broadening the explainable AI (XAI) design space by looking at explanations across the AI lifecycle. In: Proceedings of the 2021 ACM Designing Interactive Systems Conference, pp. 1591–1602. DIS '21, Association for Computing Machinery, New York, NY, USA (2021). https://doi.org/10.1145/3461778.3462131
11. Dwivedi, R., et al.: Explainable AI (XAI): core ideas, techniques, and solutions. ACM Comput. Surv. **55**(9) (2023). https://doi.org/10.1145/3561048
12. Egilmez, B., Poyraz, E., Zhou, W., Memik, G., Dinda, P., Alshurafa, N.: UStress: understanding college student subjective stress using wrist-based passive sensing. In: 2017 IEEE International Conference on Pervasive Computing and Communications Workshops (PerCom Workshops), pp. 673–678. IEEE (2017)
13. Ehsan, U., Liao, Q.V., Muller, M., Riedl, M.O., Weisz, J.D.: Expanding explainability: towards social transparency in AI systems. In: Proceedings of the 2021 CHI Conference on Human Factors in Computing Systems. CHI '21, Association for Computing Machinery, New York, NY, USA (2021). https://doi.org/10.1145/3411764.3445188
14. Epstein, D.A., Caraway, M., Johnston, C., Ping, A., Fogarty, J., Munson, S.A.: Beyond abandonment to next steps: understanding and designing for life after personal informatics tool use. In: Proceedings of the 2016 CHI Conference on Human Factors in Computing Systems, pp. 1109–1113. CHI '16, Association for Computing Machinery, New York, NY, USA (2016). https://doi.org/10.1145/2858036.2858045
15. Figueiredo, M.C., Ankrah, E., Powell, J.E., Epstein, D.A., Chen, Y.: Powered by AI: examining how AI descriptions influence perceptions of fertility tracking applications. Proc. ACM Interact. Mob. Wearable Ubiquitous Technol. **7**(4) (2024). https://doi.org/10.1145/3631414
16. Mitchell, G.E., et al.: From reflection to action: combining machine learning with expert knowledge for nutrition goal recommendations. In: Proceedings of the 2021 CHI Conference on Human Factors in Computing Systems. CHI '21, Association for Computing Machinery, New York, NY, USA (2021). https://doi.org/10.1145/3411764.3445555

17. Garcia-Ceja, E., Riegler, M., Nordgreen, T., Jakobsen, P., Oedegaard, K.J., Tørresen, J.: Mental health monitoring with multimodal sensing and machine learning: a survey. Pervasive Mob. Comput. **51**, 1–26 (2018)
18. Gleeson, M., Nieman, D.C., Pedersen, B.K.: Exercise, nutrition and immune function. Food, Nutr. Sports Perform. **II**, 186–203 (2004)
19. Gulliver, A., Griffiths, K.M., Christensen, H.: Perceived barriers and facilitators to mental health help-seeking in young people: a systematic review. BMC Psychiatry **10**(1), 1–9 (2010)
20. Haskell, W.L., et al.: Physical activity and public health: updated recommendation for adults from the American college of sports medicine and the American heart association. Circulation **116**(9), 1081 (2007)
21. Hirshkowitz, M., et al.: National sleep foundation's updated sleep duration recommendations: final report. Sleep Health **1**(4), 233–243 (2015). https://doi.org/10.1016/2015.10.004, https://www.sciencedirect.com/science/article/pii/S2352721815001606
22. Hollis, V., et al.: What does all this data mean for my future mood? Actionable analytics and targeted reflection for emotional well-being. Human-Comput. Interact. **32**(5–6), 208–267 (2017)
23. Huang, K., Sparto, P.J., Kiesler, S., Smailagic, A., Mankoff, J., Siewiorek, D.: A technology probe of wearable in-home computer-assisted physical therapy. In: Proceedings of the SIGCHI Conference on Human Factors in Computing Systems, pp. 2541–2550. CHI '14, Association for Computing Machinery, New York, NY, USA (2014). https://doi.org/10.1145/2556288.2557416
24. Hulkko, S., Mattelmäki, T., Virtanen, K., Keinonen, T.: Mobile probes. In: Proceedings of the Third Nordic Conference on Human-Computer Interaction, pp. 43–51. NordiCHI '04, Association for Computing Machinery, New York, NY, USA (2004). https://doi.org/10.1145/1028014.1028020
25. Kazi, F.F., Sandbulte, J.: Examining a social-based system with personalized recommendations to promote mental health for college students. Smart Health **28**, 100385 (2023). https://doi.org/10.1016/j.smhl.2023.100385, https://www.sciencedirect.com/science/article/pii/S2352648323000132
26. Kim, T., et al.: Prediction for retrospection: integrating algorithmic stress prediction into personal informatics systems for college students' mental health. In: CHI Conference on Human Factors in Computing Systems, pp. 1–20 (2022)
27. Kim, T., Ruensuk, M., Hong, H.: In Helping a Vulnerable Bot, You Help Yourself: Designing a Social Bot as a Care-Receiver to Promote Mental Health and Reduce Stigma, pp. 1–13. Association for Computing Machinery, New York, NY, USA (2020). https://doi.org/10.1145/3313831.3376743
28. Kitzrow, M.A.: The mental health needs of today's college students: challenges and recommendations. J. Student Aff. Res. Pract. **41**(1), 167–181 (2003)
29. Kruzan, K.P., Ng, A., Stiles-Shields, C., Lattie, E.G., Mohr, D.C., Reddy, M.: The perceived utility of smartphone and wearable sensor data in digital self-tracking technologies for mental health. In: Proceedings of the 2023 CHI Conference on Human Factors in Computing Systems. CHI '23, Association for Computing Machinery, New York, NY, USA (2023). https://doi.org/10.1145/3544548.3581209
30. Lane, N.D., et al.: BeWell: sensing sleep, physical activities and social interactions to promote wellbeing. Mob. Netw. Appl. **19**(3), 345–359 (2014)
31. Lattie, E.G., Adkins, E.C., Winquist, N., Stiles-Shields, C., Wafford, Q.E., Graham, A.K.: Digital mental health interventions for depression, anxiety, and

enhancement of psychological well-being among college students: systematic review. J. Med. Internet Res. **21**(7), e12869 (2019)
32. Lattie, E.G., Kornfield, R., Ringland, K.E., Zhang, R., Winquist, N., Reddy, M.: Designing Mental Health Technologies That Support the Social Ecosystem of College Students, pp. 1–15. Association for Computing Machinery, New York, NY, USA (2020). https://doi.org/10.1145/3313831.3376362
33. Lazar, A., Koehler, C., Tanenbaum, T.J., Nguyen, D.H.: Why we use and abandon smart devices. In: Proceedings of the 2015 ACM International Joint Conference on Pervasive and Ubiquitous Computing, pp. 635–646. UbiComp '15, Association for Computing Machinery, New York, NY, USA (2015). https://doi.org/10.1145/2750858.2804288
34. Lazar, J., Feng, J.H., Hochheiser, H.: Research methods in human-computer interaction. Morgan Kaufmann (2017)
35. Lee, K., Hong, H.: MindNavigator: exploring the stress and self-interventions for mental wellness. In: Proceedings of the 2018 CHI Conference on Human Factors in Computing Systems, pp. 1–14. CHI '18, Association for Computing Machinery, New York, NY, USA (2018). https://doi.org/10.1145/3173574.3174146
36. Liao, M., Sundar, S.S., B. Walther, J.: User trust in recommendation systems: a comparison of content-based, collaborative and demographic filtering. In: CHI Conference on Human Factors in Computing Systems, pp. 1–14 (2022)
37. Lin, Y., Jessurun, J., De Vries, B., Timmermans, H.: Motivate: towards context-aware recommendation mobile system for healthy living. In: 2011 5th International Conference on Pervasive Computing Technologies for Healthcare (PervasiveHealth) and Workshops, pp. 250–253. IEEE (2011)
38. Lu, H., et al.: StressSense: detecting stress in unconstrained acoustic environments using smartphones. In: Proceedings of the 2012 ACM Conference on Ubiquitous Computing, pp. 351–360. UbiComp '12, Association for Computing Machinery, New York, NY, USA (2012). https://doi.org/10.1145/2370216.2370270
39. Mohr, D.C., Zhang, M., Schueller, S.M.: Personal sensing: understanding mental health using ubiquitous sensors and machine learning. Annu. Rev. Clin. Psychol. **13**, 23 (2017)
40. Morshed, M.B., et al.: Prediction of mood instability with passive sensing. Proc. ACM Interact. Mob. Wearable Ubiquitous Technol. **3**(3) (2019). https://doi.org/10.1145/3351233
41. Nepal, S., et al.: COVID student study: a year in the life of college students during the COVID-19 pandemic through the lens of mobile phone sensing. In: Proceedings of the 2022 CHI Conference on Human Factors in Computing Systems, pp. 1–19 (2022)
42. Newn, J., Kelly, R.M., D'Alfonso, S., Lederman, R.: Examining and promoting explainable recommendations for personal sensing technology acceptance. Proc. ACM Interact. Mob. Wearable Ubiquitous Technol. **6**(3) (2022). https://doi.org/10.1145/3550297
43. Pedrelli, P., Nyer, M., Yeung, A., Zulauf, C., Wilens, T.: College students: mental health problems and treatment considerations. Acad. Psychiatry **39**, 503–511 (2015)
44. Saha, K., De Choudhury, M.: Assessing the mental health of college students by leveraging social media data. XRDS: Crossroads, ACM Mag. Students **28**(1), 54–58 (2021). https://doi.org/10.1145/3481834
45. Sandbulte, J., Tsai, C.H., Carroll, J.M.: Working together in a phamilySpace: facilitating collaboration on healthy behaviors over distance. Proc. ACM Hum. Comput. Interact. **5**(CSCW1) (2021). https://doi.org/10.1145/3449198

46. Sharma, A., Cosley, D.: Do social explanations work? Studying and modeling the effects of social explanations in recommender systems. In: Proceedings of the 22nd International Conference on World Wide Web, pp. 1133–1144. WWW '13, Association for Computing Machinery, New York, NY, USA (2013). https://doi.org/10.1145/2488388.2488487
47. Son, C., Hegde, S., Smith, A., Wang, X., Sasangohar, F., et al.: Effects of COVID-19 on college students' mental health in the united states: interview survey study. J. Med. Internet Res. **22**(9), e21279 (2020)
48. Center for Spirituality, Healing, E.E.B.: Wellbeing assessment (2022). https://www.takingcharge.csh.umn.edu/wellbeing-assessment. Accessed 02 Feb 2022
49. Steptoe, A., Peacey, V., Wardle, J.: Sleep duration and health in young adults. Arch. Internal Med. **166**(16), 1689–1692 (2006). https://doi.org/10.1001/archinte.166.16.1689
50. Stolzenberg, E.B., et al.: The American freshman: National norms fall 2019. Higher Education Research Institute, UCLA **42** (2020)
51. Strand, B., Roesler, K.: Calorie education: a new plan of study in physical education. J. Phys. Educ. Recreation Dance **70**(9), 46–52 (1999)
52. Su, X., Khoshgoftaar, T.M.: A survey of collaborative filtering techniques. Adv. Artif. Intell. **2009** (2009)
53. Thieme, A., Balaam, M., Wallace, J., Coyle, D., Lindley, S.: Designing wellbeing. In: Proceedings of the Designing Interactive Systems Conference, pp. 789–790 (2012)
54. Thieme, A., Wallace, J., Meyer, T.D., Olivier, P.: Designing for mental wellbeing: towards a more holistic approach in the treatment and prevention of mental illness. In: Proceedings of the 2015 British HCI Conference, pp. 1–10 (2015)
55. Velichkovska, B., Denkovski, D., Gjoreski, H., Kalendar, M., Osmani, V.: A survey of bias in healthcare: pitfalls of using biased datasets and applications. In: Computer Science On-line Conference, pp. 570–584. Springer (2023)
56. Wang, R., et al.: Tracking depression dynamics in college students using mobile phone and wearable sensing. Proc. ACM Interact. Mob. Wearable Ubiquitous Technol. **2**(1) (2018). https://doi.org/10.1145/3191775
57. Wang, X., Hegde, S., Son, C., Keller, B., Smith, A., Sasangohar, F., et al.: Investigating mental health of us college students during the COVID-19 pandemic: cross-sectional survey study. J. Med. Internet Res. **22**(9), e22817 (2020)
58. Wilks, C.R., et al.: The importance of physical and mental health in explaining health-related academic role impairment among college students. J. Psychiatr. Res. **123**, 54–61 (2020)
59. Williams, L., et al.: Analysis of distance-based mental health support for underrepresented university students. In: Extended Abstracts of the 2021 CHI Conference on Human Factors in Computing Systems. CHI EA '21, Association for Computing Machinery, New York, NY, USA (2021). https://doi.org/10.1145/3411763.3451708
60. Yoo, D.W., De Choudhury, M.: Designing dashboard for campus stakeholders to support college student mental health. In: Proceedings of the 13th EAI International Conference on Pervasive Computing Technologies for Healthcare, pp. 61–70. PervasiveHealth'19, Association for Computing Machinery, New York, NY, USA (2019). https://doi.org/10.1145/3329189.3329200
61. Zhang, J., Zhang, Q., Ai, Z., Li, X.: Context-based user typicality collaborative filtering recommendation. Hum. Centric Intell. Syst. **1**(1), 43–53 (2021)

Analysis Applications

Leveraging mHealth and Artificial Intelligence for Enhanced Health Indicators, A TwiMV Framework Proposal

Domínguez-Miranda Sergio Arturo(✉) [iD] and Rodriguez-Aguilar Roman [iD]

Facultad de Ciencias Económicas y Empresariales, Universidad Panamericana, Mexico University, Augusto Rodin 498, 03920 Mexico City, Mexico
sergioadominguezm.phd@gmail.com

Abstract. Technological advances and artificial intelligence (AI) are transforming healthcare by improving prevention, diagnosis, and remote health monitoring. This paper explores the current landscape of the potential application of digital technologies to the healthcare sector. The design of the TwiMV system is proposed to integrate diverse health data for patient diagnosis and monitoring, in a comprehensive framework, encompassing biochemical studies, genetic analysis, medical images, biometric data, dietary and lifestyle information, and wearable data. The proposal involves real-time processing through cloud-based platforms, as well as the integration of artificial intelligence algorithms and digital technologies. The proposed system aims to improve health management through personalized interventions, with specialized modules addressing priority conditions such as stroke, cardiovascular disease, oncology, diabetes, and neurological disorders.

Keywords: AI-driven Health Monitoring · Predictive Health Analytics · Digital Twin · Wearables · mHealth · Personalized Health Interventions

1 Introduction

Technological advancements have transformed healthcare, particularly in addressing non-communicable diseases (NCD) and improving health monitoring through AI integration (Dominguez-Miranda & Rodriguez-Aguilar, 2023). As global populations age and NCD become more common, technology-driven solutions are essential for enhancing health outcomes and reducing disparities.

Wearable technologies such as smartwatches, fitness trackers, and biometric sensors have revolutionized health monitoring by providing real-time data on metrics like heart rate variability, physical activity, and sleep patterns (Yang & Hsu, 2010). Devices like the Apple Watch and Fitbit use advanced technologies like electrocardiography (ECG) to detect arrhythmias and photoplethysmography (PPG) for estimating heart rate and oxygen levels (Cobos Gil, 2020). Despite accuracy challenges with ECG and PPG, these devices show great potential for personal health management and early symptom detection (Kamišalić et al., 2018). Recent studies demonstrate their effectiveness in improving patient outcomes and managing chronic conditions (Smith et al., 2021; Lee & Kim, 2022).

Innovations also include smart clothing embedded with sensors for continuous monitoring of parameters like heart rate and body temperature, especially in occupational health for real-time risk assessment (Wang, 2008). In diabetes management, electrochemical glucose sensors allow continuous blood glucose monitoring, improving glycemic control and patient outcomes (Chan et al., 2012; Xie et al., 2018). Smart clothing also shows potential for monitoring respiratory patterns and detecting early signs of distress (Liu et al., 2020; Johnson & Smith, 2023).

AI and machine learning play a crucial role in analyzing the vast data generated by these technologies. These algorithms process data from wearables, electronic health records (EHR), and genetic profiles to detect patterns and predict health outcomes. For example, machine learning models have successfully predicted physical activity and sleep quality based on wearable data (Cook et al., 2022). During the COVID-19 pandemic, AI-driven models used wearable data to predict infections with high accuracy, showcasing AI's potential in early disease detection (Hijazi et al., 2021). Further studies focus on integrating AI for enhanced disease prediction and prevention (Gupta et al., 2023; Wang & Zhang, 2024).

Recent advancements have integrated diverse health indicators into predictive models. AI-driven models now combine genetic data with lifestyle factors to predict susceptibility to chronic diseases like cardiovascular conditions and diabetes (Yun et al., 2022). Other studies explore AI in personalized medicine, tailoring treatment plans based on individual health data and genetic profiles (Hussain & Naaz, 2021; Mendhe et al., 2024).

Advances in medical imaging have also enabled AI algorithms to analyze complex images for early disease detection. Convolutional Neural Networks (CNN) are increasingly used to interpret X-rays and MRIs, providing accurate diagnostic insights and improving patient outcomes (Esteva et al., 2017; Shin et al., 2016). Recent research in oncology has highlighted AI's application in detecting early-stage cancer, improving survival rates through timely interventions (Venkatesh et al., 2021; Cheung & Rubin, 2021).

The integration of diverse health indicators into predictive models is at the forefront of research, aiming to enhance healthcare delivery by providing a comprehensive view of health status and predicting future outcomes. Genetic data reveals disease predispositions, diagnostic imaging identifies abnormalities, and real-time data from wearables offer insights into daily health fluctuations.

This research is the first step towards the development of a wearable-based digital twin for patient diagnosis and monitoring, called TwiMV (Multivariate Twin Model). The proposal contemplates an integrated system that uses artificial intelligence tools and digital technologies to analyze a wide range of health-related data. Specifically, it covers biometric data, blood chemistry, genetic information, diagnostic images, lifestyle factors, dietary habits, and real-time information collected from wearable devices. The main objective is to have predictions of the patient's health status in real time, allowing monitoring of assigned treatments and patient health outcomes. This article seeks to contribute to the evolving field of health management through the application of digital technologies. The following sections generally describe the components that will make up the TwiMV digital twin, the health indicators to be monitored, the main AI and Machine Learning (ML) tools to be used, as well as the data collection and storage mechanisms.

2 Health Indicators and Relevant Information for the TwiMV

The design of the digital twin for disease diagnosis, monitoring and prevention requires a comprehensive set of information related to the patient's health status as well as health habits. This section describes the main indicators and information to be considered in TwiMV for disease prediction and prevention.

2.1 Biometrics

Biometric information is crucial for developing predictive algorithms for disease prevention. It includes physiological and behavioral traits like heart rate, body temperature, and physical activity, offering valuable insights into health status and disease risk. Research highlights its effectiveness in monitoring and managing conditions. For instance, heart rate variability (HRV) serves as an early indicator of cardiovascular issues, facilitating timely interventions, while wearable blood pressure monitors aid in managing hypertension and reducing complications (Kleiger et al., 2005; Stergiou et al., 2018).

Biometric data also aids in metabolic condition management. Continuous glucose monitoring through wearables helps manage diabetes by enabling precise insulin dosing and lifestyle adjustments, preventing complications such as cardiovascular disease (Klonoff et al., 2017). Unlike generalized health data, biometrics reflect individual physiological variability, enabling personalized risk assessments and interventions. Combining genetic predispositions with biometric data enhances disease risk predictions, allowing for tailored prevention strategies (Hassel et al., 2015).

2.2 Blood Chemistry and Hematometric Data

Blood chemistry and hematometric data offer critical insights into metabolic, nutritional, and overall health, aiding in risk identification and disease prediction. Blood chemistry examines substances like glucose, lipids, and enzymes to assess metabolic functions. Elevated LDL cholesterol and triglycerides, for example, are major cardiovascular risk factors, with studies showing that regular monitoring improves hyperlipidemia management (Catapano et al., 2016). Blood glucose and HbA1c levels are pivotal in diabetes prevention and management, as maintaining target HbA1c levels can delay complications like nephropathy (Inzucchi et al., 2015). Predictive algorithms integrating these markers enhance diabetes progression forecasting and personalized treatment.

Hematometric data, including complete blood counts (CBCs), provide further insights. CBC abnormalities can signal anemia, infections, or malignancies; for instance, elevated white blood cell counts often indicate inflammation or infection, while low hemoglobin suggests anemia (Weiss et al., 2016). Incorporating these datasets into machine learning models enables precise disease onset prediction. By analyzing patterns across multiple biomarkers, algorithms can assess risks for cardiovascular or metabolic disorders, facilitating early intervention and tailored treatments (Obermeyer & Emanuel, 2016).

2.3 The Significance of Genetic Studies

Genetic studies are central to predictive medicine, offering key insights into inherited disease risks. Genome-wide association studies have identified genetic variants linked to conditions such as cancer, cardiovascular diseases, and metabolic disorders (Visscher et al., 2017). For instance, BRCA1 and BRCA2 mutations significantly increase breast and ovarian cancer risk, allowing for early detection through genetic testing (Lynch et al., 2016).

Incorporating genetic data into predictive algorithms enables risk stratification through polygenic risk scores (PRS), which aggregate genetic variants to estimate disease likelihood. PRS effectively predict risks for conditions like type 2 diabetes, cardiovascular diseases, and cancer, guiding tailored preventive measures (Khera et al., 2018). Understanding genetic mechanisms also drives precision medicine by identifying therapeutic targets and enabling personalized treatments, such as drugs optimized for individual metabolic profiles (Johnson et al., 2017).

Genetic data enhances early detection and monitoring. Programs like newborn screening for disorders such as phenylketonuria allow for timely interventions, preventing severe outcomes (Miller et al., 2018). Similarly, genetic testing for familial hypercholesterolemia supports early cholesterol-lowering treatments, reducing cardiovascular risks (Nordestgaard et al., 2016).

Advances in sequencing technologies and bioinformatics have expanded access to genetic data. Methods like whole-genome sequencing provide comprehensive genetic insights, while advanced computational tools improve data interpretation and integration into predictive models, increasing their clinical accuracy and utility (Mardis, 2008).

2.4 The Role of Medical Imaging

Medical imaging technologies, including CT, MRI, and ultrasound, are essential in diagnostics and preventive medicine, offering high-resolution images for early disease detection. CT scans provide precise cross-sectional views for identifying tumors and internal bleeding, while MRI excels in imaging soft tissues, aiding diagnoses of neurological disorders and certain cancers. Ultrasound, though less detailed, is widely used for real-time organ evaluation and prenatal care (Bernard, 2019; Paulson & O'Malley, 2020).

Incorporating imaging data into predictive algorithms significantly improves diagnostic accuracy. Machine learning models, particularly convolutional neural networks (CNN), excel in image analysis, detecting abnormalities like lung nodules or brain tumors with high precision (Esteva et al., 2017; Liu et al., 2019). Other algorithms, such as support vector machines and random forests, effectively classify normal versus pathological conditions, while ensemble methods enhance prediction reliability (Huang et al., 2019; Zhang et al., 2020).

Data preprocessing is critical for predictive model integration. Techniques like image normalization reduce variability, registration aligns images for accurate comparison, and augmentation generates synthetic variations to enhance model robustness (Shorten & Khoshgoftaar, 2019). For instance, deep learning models have been used to predict breast cancer from mammograms with high sensitivity and to monitor Alzheimer's progression through MRI analysis (Luo, L. et al., 2020; Yang et al., 2021).

Future advancements will focus on integrating AI and radiomics into predictive imaging models, enabling personalized risk assessments and tailored prevention based on imaging profiles. These developments promise significant strides in disease prediction and management.

2.5 Dietary Assessment and Analyzing Food Intake from Images

Dietary intake plays a critical role in overall health, significantly influencing the prevention and management of chronic diseases such as obesity, diabetes, cardiovascular disease, and cancer (Mozaffarian et al., 2016). However, traditional dietary assessment methods, like food diaries and recall interviews, are often prone to inaccuracies and biases (Slaughter et al., 2021). Machine learning has emerged as a transformative tool to enhance dietary assessment by analyzing food images, improving the precision and efficiency of dietary data collection and analysis.

Machine learning in dietary assessment relies on several key steps to enhance the accuracy and effectiveness of dietary analysis. High-quality food images are foundational to this process, with advancements in smartphone cameras and imaging software facilitating detailed image capture. Preprocessing techniques such as image enhancement and normalization further optimize image quality for analysis (Chen et al., 2019). Convolutional Neural Networks (CNN) play a critical role in feature extraction by identifying food items, portion sizes, and types with high accuracy. By learning spatial hierarchies, CNN models excel at recognizing diverse food items (Krizhevsky et al., 2012). Once features are extracted, algorithms like Support Vector Machines (SVM), Random Forests, and deep learning models classify food items and estimate their nutritional content. Combining CNN and Recurrent Neural Networks (RNN) enhances predictions by integrating visual and sequential features, as demonstrated by Zhang et al. (2020), who linked CNN-derived features with nutritional databases to estimate calorie content.

Machine learning applications in dietary management are transformative. Personalized nutrition is enabled by analyzing food images to suggest healthier alternatives, adjust portion sizes, and tailor advice to individual health goals and conditions (Liu et al., 2020). Real-time dietary monitoring allows users to track daily food intake and receive immediate feedback, empowering them to make informed dietary decisions (Kim et al., 2019). Furthermore, large-scale analysis of food images provides researchers with insights into dietary patterns and their impact on health, guiding public health strategies and interventions (Vincenzo et al., 2017). The integration of advanced machine learning models with dietary assessment tools holds immense potential for improving health outcomes. By enabling accurate, real-time analysis and personalized insights, these technologies empower individuals to adopt healthier dietary behaviors while supporting the development of effective public health initiatives.

3 Main Application of AI and ML in Disease Prediction and Prevention

Research by Domínguez-Miranda and Rodríguez-Aguilar (2024) highlights significant advancements in applying ML to health prevention, promotion, and labor productivity, with a 23.25% annual increase in related scientific output since 2008. An analysis of 87 articles underscores a focus on health-related themes and the central role of ML, particularly deep learning, in predicting and enhancing productivity. Frequent references to terms like "healthcare," "machine learning," and "prediction" reflect growing recognition of ML potential to improve health outcomes and productivity metrics.

ML algorithms such as random forests, decision trees, adaptive boosting, Bayesian methods, and neural networks are widely used, with deep learning standing out for its ability to handle large, complex datasets. This approach has proven effective in analyzing diverse health data types, including biometric, biochemical, medical imaging, wearables, and dietary information.

The findings emphasize the transformative potential of ML in addressing health and productivity challenges. The integration of ML models offers promising solutions, while ongoing research remains essential to refine these tools and expand their applications. Deep learning's prominence in contemporary research highlights its critical role in advancing health management and productivity analysis.

ML has significantly advanced the analysis of diverse health data types, including biometric, biochemical, medical imaging, lifestyle, wearables, and dietary information. This report shown in Table 1 provides an overview of various ML algorithms used in these domains, illustrating their applications and effectiveness in predicting and preventing diseases.

Table 1. Health indicators and ML algorithms

Algorithm	Domain	Focus	Reference
Support Vector Machines (SVM)	Biometric Data	Classifying high-dimensional biometric features	Cortes & Vapnik, 1995
Random Forests	Biometric Data	Improving classification accuracy with ensemble trees	Breiman, 2001
K-Nearest Neighbors (KNN)	Biometric Data	Classifying based on proximity to known samples	Cover & Hart, 1967
Principal Component Analysis (PCA)	Biochemical Data	Reducing dimensionality and identifying patterns	Jolliffe, 1986

(*continued*)

Table 1. (*continued*)

Algorithm	Domain	Focus	Reference
Logistic Regression	Biochemical Data	Modeling probability of disease presence	Hosmer & Lemeshow, 2000
Gradient Boosting Machines (GBM)	Biochemical Data	Enhancing performance through boosting	Friedman, 2001
Convolutional Neural Networks (CNN)	Medical Imaging	Classifying and detecting abnormalities in images	LeCun et al., 1998
U-Net	Medical Imaging	Segmenting structures in biomedical images	Ronneberger et al., 2015
Generative Adversarial Networks (GAN)	Medical Imaging	Generating synthetic images and enhancing quality	Goodfellow et al., 2014
Decision Trees	Lifestyle Information	Classifying lifestyle-related data with decision rules	Breiman et al., 1986
Naive Bayes	Lifestyle Information	Predicting outcomes based on lifestyle attributes	Rennie et al., 2003
K-Means Clustering	Lifestyle Information	Grouping individuals based on lifestyle factors	MacQueen, 1967
Long Short-Term Memory (LSTM) Networks	Wearables	Analyzing time-series data for pattern detection	Hochreiter & Schmidhuber, 1997
Hidden Markov Models (HMM)	Wearables	Modeling sequential data and detecting transitions	Rabiner, 1989
Autoencoders	Wearables	Learning efficient representations for anomaly detection	Hinton & Salakhutdinov, 2006
Convolutional Neural Networks (CNN)	Dietary Intake	Classifying and tracking food items from images	Krizhevsky et al., 2012

(*continued*)

Table 1. (*continued*)

Algorithm	Domain	Focus	Reference
Deep Learning Architectures	Dietary Intake	Enhancing recognition with deep network structures	He et al., 2016; Huang et al., 2017
Image Segmentation Techniques	Dietary Intake	Detecting and segmenting food items in images	He et al., 2017

4 Wearable Devices

Wearable devices have become a transformative tool in health monitoring, providing real-time data for predictive analytics in disease prevention and management. These devices track various health metrics, such as heart rate, physical activity, sleep patterns, and body temperature, offering valuable insights into an individual's health. For instance, changes in heart rate or sleep quality can signal potential health issues like cardiovascular problems or metabolic disorders (Horsfall et al., 2021; Pino et al., 2022).

One key application of wearables is in the early detection of health conditions. Machine learning algorithms analyze wearable data to identify patterns that signal diseases such as diabetes, hypertension, or arrhythmias. For example, heart rate variability data from wearables has been used to predict cardiovascular events (Zhao et al., 2019). Wearable data also aids in managing conditions like obesity and insomnia (Hafner et al., 2019). Additionally, wearables enable personalized health management by integrating real-time data with other factors like genetics and lifestyle, offering tailored recommendations (Doherty et al., 2018; Zhan et al., 2021).

The integration of wearables with other health technologies, such as electronic health records (EHR) and telemedicine, enhances predictive analytics. Combining wearable data with clinical information allows for more accurate predictions and better healthcare decisions (McCormack et al., 2019; Sierksma et al., 2020). Wearables also contribute to public health monitoring, with aggregated data helping identify trends across populations and evaluate public health interventions (Cowan et al., 2019; Li et al., 2022).

4.1 The Role of Questionnaires and Applications

Lifestyle factors, such as smoking, alcohol consumption, and physical activity, significantly influence health outcomes, affecting conditions like cardiovascular diseases, respiratory disorders, and metabolic syndrome (World Health Organization, 2021). Accurately assessing these factors is crucial for predictive analytics, enabling the identification of high-risk individuals and the implementation of targeted interventions.

Questionnaires are commonly used to collect information on lifestyle factors, capturing data on smoking habits, alcohol intake, physical activity levels, and other behaviors. Tools like the Global Physical Activity Questionnaire assess physical activity patterns, while the Fagerström Test for Nicotine Dependence measures nicotine dependence (Pope et al., 2020; Heatherton et al., 1991). These questionnaires can be integrated with machine learning models to predict health risks, allowing for early intervention and personalized recommendations (Choi et al., 2020).

Mobile applications have gained popularity in monitoring lifestyle factors, offering real-time data collection and user-friendly interfaces. Apps like MyFitnessPal and Fitbit track physical activity, dietary intake, and health metrics, often integrating with wearable devices for continuous monitoring (Patrick et al., 2016). Other apps, such as AlcoDroid and Drinkaware, help monitor and reduce alcohol consumption, providing insights into drinking patterns and supporting personalized intervention strategies (Haug et al., 2013). Data from these apps can enhance predictive models and inform health recommendations based on individual behaviors.

5 Methodological Framework of TwiMV Development

According to the health indicators and relevant information considered, the components of the TwiMV information integration module are presented in Table 2. The objective is to have a comprehensive view of information on the patient's health status and habits.

The proposed architecture for TwiMV is presented in Fig. 1, which shows the integration and use of various types of health data for predictive analysis. This diagram aims to visually represent the various sources of information and their inter-connections, highlighting how they collectively contribute to the development of advanced predictive models in health. By integrating these various components, the design underscores the potential for creating a robust predictive model that leverages comprehensive health data to improve individual and organizational health out-comes.

In the proposed system, the transformation of various health-related variables into actionable insights is achieved through the application of advanced mathematical algorithms and cloud-based technologies. The process involves several key stages, each utilizing state-of-the-art methods to handle and analyze the diverse types of data collected. The analysis of a set of selected diseases will be integrated through specialized modules as shown in Fig. 1. It is worth mentioning the integration of a labor module that will collect the effect of the patient's health status on his/her work productivity. This module will be integrated according to the specific needs of the users. A critical path was considered for the implementation of TwiMV, according to the stages established in Table 3.

The transformed data in the TwiMV system will be utilized to achieve several key objectives, including individual characterization, data visualization, intelligent health prediction, preventive measures, and integrating Value-Based Healthcare (VBHC) principles to assess cost-effectiveness. Each of these elements leverages advanced algorithms and technologies to provide a comprehensive health management solution.

- **Individual Characterization** is achieved through the application of Principal Component Analysis (PCA) and Index Generation techniques. PCA reduces the dimensionality of complex health data by identifying significant components that explain the variance in the data, simplifying the representation of an individual's health profile for easier interpretation and analysis. Additionally, custom indices are generated

Table 2. Indicators and information that will feed TwiMV

Component	Description
Biochemical Studies	Involves hematological profiles and blood chemistry analyses, providing essential metrics (e.g., red/white blood cell counts, hemoglobin levels) and insights into metabolic functions
Genetic Studies	Focuses on traits, mutations, and predispositions, integrating data on genetic variants and their associations with health conditions to assess susceptibility to diseases
Medical Imaging Studies	Includes imaging modalities (e.g., CT scans, MRI, ultrasound) that provide detailed visual information on internal structures, essential for diagnosis and monitoring health issues
Biometric Data	Covers biometric measurements (e.g., body mass, body fat percentage) that offer insights into physical health and fitness levels, integral to understanding overall well-being
Dietary Information	Utilizes data from food photographs and dietary questionnaires to analyze nutritional intake and its impact on health, evaluating eating habits and health outcomes
Lifestyle Information	Derived from questionnaires and voice recordings, capturing lifestyle habits (e.g., smoking, alcohol consumption, physical activity) to understand their influence on health
Wearable Device Data	Integrates data from wearable technology (e.g., smart bracelets, glucose meters) for continuous health monitoring, providing real-time insights into various health metrics

to encapsulate various health metrics into a single composite measure, integrating biometric data, biochemical markers, lifestyle factors, and other relevant variables to provide a holistic view of an individual's health status.
- **Data Visualization** plays a crucial role in interpreting health information and tracking individual progress. The system employs advanced dashboards and mobile applications to present data in an accessible and actionable format. Interactive dashboards allow users to view general population statistics, including average health metrics and distributions, and make comparisons between an individual's health status and population benchmarks. This comparative analysis aids in identifying deviations and trends, facilitating personalized health management strategies.
- **Intelligent Health Prediction** is realized through various machine learning algorithms. Neural networks, including deep learning models, analyze complex patterns to make accurate predictions about health outcomes. For instance, CNN is used to analyze medical images, while RNN manage time-series data from wearables. K-Means clustering groups individuals with similar health profiles for targeted interventions, and Random Forests and GBM predict disease risk and health outcomes based on multiple variables, ensuring robust and reliable predictions.
- **Prevention Through Alerts** is a key component of the system, providing real-time alerts based on detected anomalies and risk factors. Outlier detection algorithms

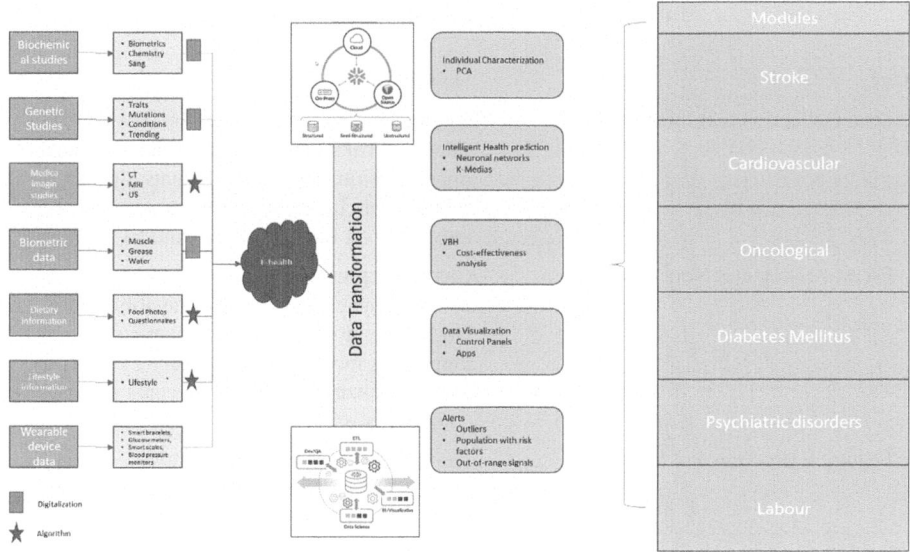

Fig. 1. TwinMV health indicators and relevant information integration

identify data points outside normal ranges, flagging potential health issues requiring attention. Risk factors and warning signals are monitored continuously, generating alerts for conditions exceeding predefined thresholds. For example, sudden spikes in glucose levels or abnormal heart rate patterns trigger notifications to users, prompting timely interventions and consultations.
- **Value-Based Healthcare (VBHC) Analysis** evaluates cost-effectiveness and optimizes healthcare delivery. This analysis involves calculating the value derived from healthcare interventions relative to their cost. The system assesses the economic impact of various health strategies by comparing the costs of preventive measures, treatments, and interventions against the achieved health outcomes. This provides insights into the most effective and cost-efficient approaches to health management, ensuring resources are allocated to interventions that deliver the greatest value in improving patient health.

Specialized analytical modules will be developed to comprehensively address various health conditions and support productivity enhancement among workers. Each module will focus on specific health concerns, leveraging the transformed data from biometric, biochemical, genetic, imaging, lifestyle, and wearable sources. These modules will be designed to provide detailed insights and actionable recommendations tailored to each health domain. Below, we outline potential modules and the relevant variables for analysis according with Table 4.

Each module will leverage advanced analytics and machine learning algorithms to analyze the relevant variables, providing targeted insights and actionable recommendations for improving health outcomes and productivity. The data collection process is illustrated in Fig. 2. It shows how integrating data from various sources and applying advanced analytical techniques enables the system to support proactive health management.

Table 3. Stages of Data Processing in TwiMV

Stage	Description
1. Data Collection and Integration	Aggregate data from various sources (biochemical studies, genetic analyses, medical imaging, biometric measurements, dietary information, lifestyle data, wearable devices) into a unified format for multimodal learning
2. Preprocessing and Normalization	Clean and preprocess data to remove inconsistencies and ensure compatibility. Normalize biochemical and genetic data, preprocess medical images to enhance quality, and normalize wearable device data for consistency
3. Feature Extraction and Selection	Identify and isolate relevant attributes from processed data, reducing dimensionality. Use CNN for medical images, PCA for genetic data, SVM and Random Forests for biometric data, and deep learning models for dietary images
4. Algorithm Application	a. **Biochemical and Genetic Data**: PCA, GBM
	b. **Medical Imaging**: CNN, U-Net
	c. **Biometric Data**: SVM, Random Forests
	d. **Dietary Information**: Deep Learning (Res-Net, DenseNet)
	e. **Lifestyle Information**: Decision Trees, Naive Bayes
	f. **Wearable Device Data**: LSTM, HMM
5. Real-Time Processing and Cloud-Based Analysis	Perform data processing and analysis in real-time using cloud platforms, enabling scalability and efficient handling of large data volumes
6. Continuous Learning and Adaptation	Incorporate continuous learning mechanisms to adapt algorithms based on new data, periodically retraining machine learning models to maintain accuracy and relevance
7. Visualization and Reporting	Present analyzed data through dashboards and visualizations, providing actionable insights for health status and productivity, facilitating informed decision-making

The health management process begins with **Data Collection and Integration**, which encompasses a multifaceted approach to gather comprehensive health information. Intelligent applications capture dietary intake and nutritional patterns through food photographs, while wearable devices monitor physiological metrics such as heart

Table 4. Summary of Health Modules and Key Variables

Module	Data Type	Key Variables
Stroke Analysis Module	Biometric	Blood pressure measurements, BMI, waist circumference
	Biochemical	Cholesterol levels, glucose levels, inflammation markers
	Genetic	Genetic predispositions to stroke-related conditions (e.g., clotting disorders)
	Imaging	Brain scan results (CT, MRI) identifying ischemic or hemorrhagic lesions
	Lifestyle	Smoking history, alcohol consumption, physical activity levels
	Wearable	Continuous monitoring of blood pressure and heart rate variability
Cardiovascular Disease Module	Biometric	Blood pressure, BMI, heart rate
	Biochemical	Lipid profiles, glucose levels, cardiac stress markers (e.g., troponin)
	Genetic	Risk-associated genetic variants (e.g., hypertension, atherosclerosis)
	Imaging	Echocardiograms, cardiac MRIs, coronary angiograms
	Lifestyle	Dietary habits, exercise routines, smoking status
	Wearable	Heart rate monitors, activity trackers
Oncology Module	Biometric	Body measurements indicating tumor growth
	Biochemical	Tumor markers, blood counts, metabolic profiles
	Genetic	Genetic mutations associated with cancer susceptibility (e.g., BRCA1/2)
	Imaging	Mammograms, PET scans, biopsies
	Lifestyle	History of carcinogen exposure, diet, physical activity
	Wearable	Monitoring activity levels, physiological responses to treatment
Diabetes Mellitus Module	Biometric	BMI, waist circumference, body fat percentage

(*continued*)

Table 4. (*continued*)

Module	Data Type	Key Variables
	Biochemical	Blood glucose levels, HbA1c, insulin sensitivity markers
	Genetic	Genetic predispositions to diabetes (e.g., glucose metabolism variants)
	Imaging	Fat distribution imaging to assess visceral fat levels
	Lifestyle	Dietary intake, physical activity levels, carbohydrate consumption history
	Wearable	Continuous glucose monitoring, activity trackers
Neurological Disorders Module	Biometric	Neurological assessments (e.g., reflexes, motor functions)
	Biochemical	Markers of neuroinflammation, neurodegeneration
	Genetic	Genetic risk factors for neurodegenerative diseases (e.g., APOE for Alzheimer's)
	Imaging	MRI and CT scans detecting brain lesions or structural changes
	Lifestyle	Cognitive activity, stress levels, sleep patterns
	Wearable	Devices monitoring sleep quality and cognitive performance
Productivity Enhancement Module	Biometric	Overall health metrics (e.g., BMI, physical fitness indicators)
	Biochemical	Wellness indicators (e.g., stress hormones, fatigue markers)
	Genetic	Genetic factors influencing work-related stress and productivity
	Imaging	Assessments of physical health impacting productivity
	Lifestyle	Work habits, stress levels, overall lifestyle balance
	Wearable	Activity trackers, stress monitors, wellness devices

rate, step count, and activity levels. This combination of data sources builds a holistic health profile for each individual and supports continuous health monitoring in line with mHealth principles.

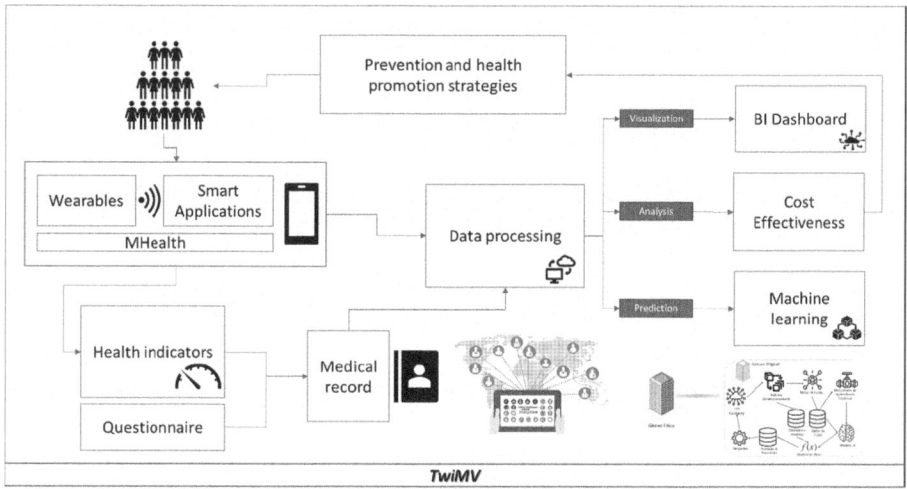

Fig. 2. TwiMV data processing

Once collected, the data is securely stored in a **Storage and Management** phase, where it is compiled into a centralized repository. This health information hub consolidates real-time indicators, including heart rate variability, physical activity levels, and dietary intake. The repository further integrates data from lifestyle questionnaires, imaging studies like CT scans and MRIs, as well as laboratory tests such as blood chemistry and hematological profiles, resulting in a cohesive medical profile for each person.

Following storage, the data undergoes a rigorous **Data Processing** phase that encompasses three key aspects:

- **Visualization.** During the visualization stage, interactive dashboards and control panels graphically represent health metrics, allowing users to view trends and compare their data against population benchmarks.
- **Advanced analytics.** Conducted to assess the economic impact of different health interventions, helping to evaluate the financial implications of preventive measures and treatments.
- **Prediction.** Machine learning analyze patterns within the data to forecast potential health issues and identify at-risk individuals. These predictive models generate actionable insights that inform targeted interventions and personalized health recommendations.

The insights gained from the visualization, analysis, and prediction phases are then utilized to develop comprehensive **Strategy Development** for health prevention and promotion. Strategies are tailored both for the general population, focusing on broad public health initiatives, and for individuals, offering personalized recommendations based on their unique health profiles.

The final stage of the process involves a feedback loop, where the outcomes and effectiveness of the implemented strategies are monitored and assessed. This continuous evaluation helps refine and optimize health recommendations and interventions. The feedback collected is used to update and enhance the data collection processes, ensuring that the system remains dynamic and responsive to evolving health needs.

6 Discussions and Conclusions

The integration of digital technologies for prevention and healthcare is a reality. However, a transition process towards the implementation of such technologies is required, as part of a digital transformation process in the healthcare sector. The digital transition will allow for more precise and personalized health interventions by analyzing various data sources. This integration facilitates a comprehensive understanding of individual health profiles, leading to more effective prevention and management strategies. An additional benefit is the potential improvement in work productivity. By proactively addressing health issues and optimizing health management strategies, companies can improve employee well-being and productivity. Employers benefit from reduced healthcare costs and absenteeism, while employees experience better health outcomes and job satisfaction.

Despite these benefits, the research identified several challenges such as the integration and analysis of various data sources. The combination of biometric data, biochemical profiles, genetic information, imaging results, and lifestyle factors re-quires sophisticated data management and processing capabilities. Ensuring the accuracy, privacy, and security of these is paramount, given the sensitive nature of health information. Another challenge is the need for ongoing validation and refinement of machine learning models. While these algorithms are promising, their effectiveness depends on the quality and representativeness of the data they are trained on. Ongoing validation is necessary to ensure that models remain accurate and reliable over time. Furthermore, the changing nature of health data and medical knowledge requires regular updates to predictive algorithms and models to maintain their relevance and effectiveness. Implementing machine learning-driven health strategies in real-world settings poses logistical and ethical challenges. Translating predictive insights into viable health interventions requires careful consideration of ethical implications. There is a need for interdisciplinary collaboration to bridge the gap between data science, healthcare, and policymaking to ensure that machine learning applications are used responsibly and effectively.

The design of the TwiMV integrates multiple data sources to be able to provide a holistic view of an individual's health. This approach is crucial for developing de-tailed health profiles and personalized prevention strategies. Real-time processing and visualization of integrated data through cloud-based ML solutions further enables dynamic monitoring and immediate feedback. Tools such as dashboards and mobile apps play a key role in presenting this data in an accessible format, allowing people to compare their health metrics to population benchmarks and make in-formed health decisions. The feasibility, limitations, and expected outcomes of the TwiMV framework, along with the development process, inputs, methods, and target population, should be discussed. Future lines of research have already been identified, including evaluating the efficacy of the TwiMV framework across diverse demographic groups, exploring integration with telehealth services to enhance remote monitoring, and assessing user engagement and adherence to recommended interventions. Additionally, including empirical data or pilot studies demonstrating the feasibility and real-world application of the TwiMV framework would provide valuable insights into its practical utility.

References

Bernard, J.: Medical imaging technologies and their applications in clinical practice. Med. Imaging Rev. **29**(2), 123–135 (2019). https://doi.org/10.1016/j.mir.2018.10.002

Breiman, L., Friedman, J., Olshen, R.A., Stone, C.J.: Classification and regression trees. Chapman & Hall (1986). https://doi.org/10.1201/9781315139470

Breiman, L.: Random forests. Mach. Learn. **45**(1), 5–32 (2001). https://doi.org/10.1023/A:1010933404324

Chan, S.Y., Woon, C.S.: Glucose monitoring in diabetes management: the role of continuous glucose monitoring. J. Diabetes Sci. Technol. **6**(2), 487–491 (2012). https://doi.org/10.1177/193229681200600228

Chen, M., Ma, H., Li, T.: Image preprocessing techniques for food image analysis: a review. J. Food Sci. Technol. **56**(11), 5071–5081 (2019). https://doi.org/10.1007/s11483-019-00123-w

Cheung, H.M.C., Rubin, D.: Challenges and opportunities for artificial intelligence in oncological imaging. Clin. Radiol. **76**(10), 728–736 (2021). https://doi.org/10.1016/j.crad.2021.03.009

Choi, S., Han, K., Kim, J.: Predicting health risks using machine learning models with questionnaire data. Comput. Math. Methods Med. **2020**, 8254819 (2020). https://doi.org/10.1155/2020/8254819

Cobos Gil, M.A.: Photoplethysmography (PPG) for cardiovascular health monitoring: principles and applications. Sensors **20**(23), 6710 (2020). https://doi.org/10.3390/s20236710

Cook, D.J., Su, M.: Predicting physical activity and sleep quality using wearable data. J. Biomed. Inform. **124**, 103981 (2022). https://doi.org/10.1016/j.jbi.2021.103981

Cortes, C., Vapnik, V.: Support-vector networks. Mach. Learn. **20**(3), 273–297 (1995). https://doi.org/10.1007/BF00994018

Cover, T.M., Hart, P.E.: Nearest-neighbor pattern classification. IEEE Trans. Inf. Theory **13**(1), 21–27 (1967). https://doi.org/10.1109/TIT.1967.1053964

Cowan, L., Donnelly, P., Garcia, L.: Public health monitoring using aggregated wearable device data. Public Health Rep. **134**(3), 346–356 (2019). https://doi.org/10.1177/0033354919847022

Doherty, A., Jackson, D., McCarthy, S.: Personalized health recommendations based on wearable device data. Digital Health **4**, 1–12 (2018). https://doi.org/10.1177/2055207618780102

Dominguez-Miranda, S.A., Rodríguez-Aguilar, R.: Health 4.0, prevention, and health promotion in companies: systematic literature review. In: Computer Science and Engineering in Health Services: 6th EAI International Conference Proceedings, COMPSE 2022, Mexico City, July 28, 2022 (p. 217). Springer International Publishing (2023). https://doi.org/10.1007/978-3-031-34750-4_13

Domínguez-Miranda, S.A., Rodriguez-Aguilar, R.: Machine learning models in health prevention and promotion and labor productivity: a co-word analysis. Iberoamerican J. Sci. Measur. Commun. **4**(1), 1–16 (2024). https://doi.org/10.47909/ijsmc.85

Esteva, A., Kuprel, B., Novoa, R.A., Ko, J., Swetter, S.M., Martinez, B.: Dermatologist-level classification of skin cancer with deep neural networks. Nature **542**(7639), 115–118 (2017). https://doi.org/10.1038/nature21056

Friedman, J.H.: Greedy function approximation: a gradient boosting machine. Ann. Stat. **29**(5), 1189–1232 (2001). https://doi.org/10.1214/aos/1013203451

Goodfellow, I., et al.: Generative adversarial nets. Adv. Neural Inf. Process. Syst. **27** (2014). https://arxiv.org/abs/1406.2661

Gupta, S., Kumar, A., Singh, P.: Integrating AI in multimodal data analysis for disease prediction: a systematic review. Artif. Intell. Med. **47**, 101–115 (2023). https://doi.org/10.1016/j.artmed.2023.101115

Hafner, M., Gernsbacher, M., Schur, C.: Using wearable devices to predict and manage obesity and sleep disorders. Int. J. Obes. **43**(7), 1304–1316 (2019). https://doi.org/10.1038/s41366-019-0310-x

Hassel, S., Müller, A., Pahl, M.: The integration of biometric data into predictive health management. J. Personalized Med. **5**(3), 376–391 (2015). https://doi.org/10.3390/jpm5030376

Haug, S., Paz Castro, R., Schuster, R.: Mobile apps for alcohol use: a systematic review. Addict. Res. Theory **21**(3), 239–248 (2013). https://doi.org/10.3109/16066359.2012.748153

He, K., Zhang, X., Ren, S., Sun, J.: Deep residual learning for image recognition. In: Proceedings of the IEEE Conference on Computer Vision and Pattern Recognition (pp. 770–778) (2016). https://doi.org/10.1109/CVPR.2016.90

He, K., Zhang, X., Ren, S., Sun, J.: Mask R-CNN. In: Proceedings of the IEEE International Conference on Computer Vision, pp. 2961–2969 (2017). https://doi.org/10.1109/ICCV.2017.322

Heatherton, T.F., Kozlowski, L.T., Frecker, R.C., Fagerström, K.-O.: The Fagerström test for nicotine dependence: a revision of the Fagerström tolerance questionnaire. Br. J. Addict. **86**(9), 1119–1127 (1991). https://doi.org/10.1111/j.1360-0443.1991.tb01879.x

Hijazi, Z., Oldgren, J.: Machine learning in predicting COVID-19 infections using wearable data. Nat. Med. **27**(3), 379–385 (2021). https://doi.org/10.1038/s41591-020-01185-1

Hinton, G.E., Salakhutdinov, R.R.: Reducing the dimensionality of data with neural networks. Science **313**(5786), 504–507 (2006). https://doi.org/10.1126/science.1127647

Hochreiter, S., Schmidhuber, J.: Long short-term memory. Neural Comput. **9**(8), 1735–1780 (1997). https://doi.org/10.1162/neco.1997.9.8.1735

Horsfall, J.R., Patel, S., Khan, A.: Wearable health monitoring systems and their application in predictive analytics. J. Health Inf. **34**(3), 301–311 (2021). https://doi.org/10.1080/13551907.2021.1910359

Hosmer, D.W., Lemeshow, S.: Applied logistic regression (2nd ed.). Wiley (2000). https://doi.org/10.1002/9781118548387

Huang, G., Liu, Z., van der Maaten, L., Weinberger, K.Q.: Densely connected convolutional networks. In: Proceedings of the IEEE Conference on Computer Vision and Pattern Recognition, pp. 4700–4708 (2017). https://doi.org/10.1109/CVPR.2017.243

Huang, Y., Xu, Z., Zhao, Y., Zhang, H.: Support vector machine and random forest for classification of medical imaging data. Comput. Biol. Chem. **80**, 317–327 (2019). https://doi.org/10.1016/j.compbiolchem.2019.02.005

Hussain, A., Naaz, S.: Use of deep learning in personalized medicine: current trends and the future perspective. ICIDSSD **2020**, 21 (2021). https://doi.org/10.4108/eai.27-2-2020.2303118

Inzucchi, S.E., Bergenstal, R.M.: Management of hyperglycemia in type 2 diabetes, 2015: a patient-centered approach. Diabetes Care **38**(1), 140–149 (2015). https://doi.org/10.2337/dc14-2441

Johnson, J.A., Veenstra, D.L.: Personalized medicine: a revolution in drug therapy. Clin. Pharmacol. Ther. **101**(6), 800–809 (2017). https://doi.org/10.1002/cpt.750

Jolliffe, I.T.: Principal component analysis. Springer Series in Statistics. Springer (1986). https://doi.org/10.1007/978-1-4757-1904-8

Kamišalić, A., Herout, J.: Accuracy of ECG and PPG-based heart rate monitors: a review. Biomed. Eng. Online **17**(1), 16 (2018). https://doi.org/10.1186/s12938-018-0430-7

Khera, A.V., Chasman, D.I., Emdin, C.A.: Genetic risk, adherence to a healthy lifestyle, and coronary disease. N. Engl. J. Med. **375**(24), 2349–2358 (2018). https://doi.org/10.1056/NEJMoa1616338

Kim, J., Lee, S., Park, Y.: Real-time dietary monitoring using food image analysis and machine learning. J. Food Sci. **84**(6), 1843–1852 (2019). https://doi.org/10.1111/1750-3841.14663

Kleiger, R.E., Miller, J.P., Bigger, J.T.: Heart rate variability: measurement and clinical utility. Ann. Noninvasive Electrocardiol. **10**(1), 88–99 (2005). https://doi.org/10.1111/j.1542-474X.2005.10101.x

Klonoff, D.C., Ahn, D., Drincic, A.: Continuous glucose monitoring: a review of the technology and clinical use. Diabetes Res. Clin. Pract. **133**, 178–192 (2017). https://doi.org/10.1016/j.diabres.2017.08.005

Krizhevsky, A., Sutskever, I., Hinton, G.E.: ImageNet classification with deep convolutional neural networks. Commun. ACM **60**(6), 84–90 (2012). https://doi.org/10.1145/3065386

LeCun, Y., Bottou, L., Orr, G. B., Müller, K.-R.: Efficient backprop. In: Neural Networks: Tricks of the Trade, pp. 9–50. Springer (1998). https://doi.org/10.1007/978-3-662-03680-8_2

Lee, S., Kim, D.: Smart clothing for real-time health monitoring in occupational health settings. Occup. Health Sci. **45**(1), 89–102 (2022). https://doi.org/10.1002/ohs.23456

Li, X., Wang, Y., Chen, Z.: Aggregated data from wearables for public health monitoring and intervention. Int. J. Environ. Res. Public Health **19**(5), 2567 (2022). https://doi.org/10.3390/ijerph19052567

Liu, Y., Chen, P.H.C., Zheng, Y., de Oliveira, G.: Deep learning for detecting lung cancer from CT images: a review and future directions. J. Med. Imaging **6**(3), 1–14 (2019). https://doi.org/10.1117/1.JMI.6.3.031501

Liu, Z., Li, Z., Wang, Y., Wang, W.: Personalized nutrition recommendations based on food image analysis. J. Nutr. Sci. **9**, e17 (2020). https://doi.org/10.1017/jns.2020.12

Lynch, H.T., Snyder, C.L.: BRCA1 and BRCA2 mutations and cancer risk: a review of recent data. Breast Cancer Res. Treat. **155**(1), 1–14 (2016). https://doi.org/10.1007/s10549-015-3713-2

MacQueen, J.: Some methods for classification and analysis of multivariate observations. In: Proceedings of the Fifth Berkeley Symposium on Mathematical Statistics and Probability, (pp. 281–297). University of California Press (1967). https://projecteuclid.org/euclid.bsmsp/1200512992

Mardis, E.R.: Next-generation DNA sequencing methods. Annu. Rev. Genomics Hum. Genet. **9**(1), 387–402 (2008). https://doi.org/10.1146/annurev.genom.9.081307.164359

McCormack, R., Brown, T., Lee, M.: Enhancing predictive analytics in healthcare with wearable devices and EHR integration. Health Inform. J. **25**(2), 300–313 (2019). https://doi.org/10.1177/1460458218779752

Mendhe, D., et al.: AI-enabled data-driven approaches for personalized medicine and healthcare analytics. In: 2024 Ninth International Conference on Science Technology Engineering and Mathematics (ICONSTEM), (pp. 1–5). IEEE (2024). https://doi.org/10.1109/ICONSTEM60960.2024.10568722

Miller, D.T., Lee, K.M.: Newborn screening for genetic disorders: clinical and cost-effectiveness. J. Pediatr. **198**, 67–73 (2018). https://doi.org/10.1016/j.jpeds.2018.02.003

Miotto, R., Wang, F., Wang, S., Jiang, X., Dudley, J.T.: Deep learning for healthcare: review, opportunities and challenges. Brief. Bioinform. **19**(6), 1236–1246 (2017). https://doi.org/10.1093/bib/bbx044

Nordestgaard, B.G., Chapman, M.J.: Familial hypercholesterolemia: a review of current guidelines and future perspectives. Eur. Heart J. **37**(42), 2970–2981 (2016). https://doi.org/10.1093/eurheartj/ehw095

Obermeyer, Z., Emanuel, E.J.: Predicting the future — big data, machine learning, and clinical medicine. N. Engl. J. Med. **375**(13), 1216–1219 (2016). https://doi.org/10.1056/NEJMp1606181

Patrick, K., Raab, F., Adams, M.A.: Mobile health technology for behavioral intervention: a systematic review. J. Behav. Med. **39**(3), 405–424 (2016). https://doi.org/10.1007/s10865-016-9757-2

Paulson, E.K., O'Malley, M.: Advances in imaging technology and its impact on diagnosis and treatment. Radiol. J. **52**(4), 345–359 (2020). https://doi.org/10.1148/radiol.2020200412

Pino, J., Oliveira, C., Gozal, D.: Advanced wearable devices for health monitoring and disease prevention: a review. Sensors **22**(4), 1125 (2022). https://doi.org/10.3390/s22041125

Pope, D., Fisher, A., Smith, C.: Validation of health-related questionnaires for predictive analytics. J. Epidemiol. Community Health **74**(5), 450–459 (2020). https://doi.org/10.1136/jech-2019-213543

Rabiner, L.R.: A tutorial on hidden Markov models and selected applications in speech recognition. Proc. IEEE **77**(2), 257–286 (1989). https://doi.org/10.1109/5.18626

Rennie, J.D., Shih, L.H., Teevan, J., Karger, D.R.: Tackling the poor assumptions of Naive Bayes text classifiers. In: Proceedings of the 20th International Conference on Machine Learning, pp. 616–623 (2003). https://doi.org/10.5555/645530.655813

Ronneberger, O., Fischer, P., Brox, T.: U-Net: convolutional networks for biomedical image segmentation. In: Medical Image Computing and Computer-Assisted Intervention – MICCAI 2015, pp. 234–241. Springer (2015). https://doi.org/10.1007/978-3-319-24574-4_28

Shin, H., Roth, H., Gao, M.: Deep convolutional neural networks for computer-aided detection: CNN architectures, dataset characteristics, and transfer learning. IEEE Trans. Med. Imaging **35**(5), 1285–1298 (2016). https://doi.org/10.1109/TMI.2016.2528162

Shorten, C., Khoshgoftaar, T.M.: A survey on image data augmentation for deep learning. J. Big Data **6**(1), 1–48 (2019). https://doi.org/10.1186/s40537-019-0197-0

Sierksma, A., Schoen, M., Hoekstra, A.: Wearables and telemedicine: Enhancing health monitoring with integrated technologies. Telemedicine e-Health **26**(6), 733–740 (2020). https://doi.org/10.1089/tmj.2019.0198

Smith, L., Brown, L., Johnson, T.: The impact of wearable devices on patient outcomes: a systematic review. Health Technol. Res. **33**(4), 221–235 (2021). https://doi.org/10.1177/HTA3304020123

Stergiou, G.S., Markou, A.: Wearable devices for continuous blood pressure monitoring: a review. J. Hypertens. **36**(1), 51–60 (2018). https://doi.org/10.1097/HJH.0000000000001465

Venkadesh, K.V., et al.: Deep learning for malignancy risk estimation of pulmonary nodules detected at low-dose screening CT. Radiology **300**(2), 438–447 (2021). https://doi.org/10.1148/radiol.2021204433

Vincenzo, D., Patel, S., George, A.: Machine learning applications in dietary pattern analysis: a review. Public Health Nutr. **20**(2), 339–348 (2017). https://doi.org/10.1017/S136898001602359

Visscher, P.M., Wray, N.R.: The contributions of genetic variation to complex traits. Nature **551**(7678), 332–338 (2017). https://doi.org/10.1038/nature24371

Luo, L., et al.: Deep learning in breast cancer imaging: a decade of progress and future directions. IEEE Rev. Biomed. Eng. (2024). https://doi.org/10.1109/RBME.2024.3357877

Wang, H., Liu, X., Li, Y., Yang, Y.: Food image analysis with deep learning: a review. In: Proceedings of the IEEE Conference on Computer Vision and Pattern Recognition (pp. 1223–1232) (2018). https://doi.org/10.1109/CVPR.2018.00131

Wang, J.: Smart clothing and wearable sensors: applications and implications. J. Occup. Environ. Hyg. **5**(8), 487–495 (2008). https://doi.org/10.1080/15459620802280078

Wang, L., Zhang, S., Liu, X., Zhang, Z.: Deep learning-based prediction of breast cancer risk from mammographic images. Breast Cancer Res. **22**(1), 1–12 (2020). https://doi.org/10.1186/s13058-020-01340-8

Weiss, G., Goodnough, L.T.: Anemia of chronic disease. N. Engl. J. Med. **374**(4), 349–356 (2016). https://doi.org/10.1056/NEJMra1514144

WHO. Global physical activity questionnaire (GPAQ) analysis guide. World Health Organization (2005). https://www.who.int/publications/i/item/9789241599979

World Health Organization. Global status report on noncommunicable diseases 2021. World Health Organization (2021). https://www.who.int/publications/i/item/9789240062810

Xie, L., Reddy, T.S.: Continuous glucose monitoring: a comprehensive review. Diabetes Technol. Ther. **20**(2), 118–125 (2018). https://doi.org/10.1089/dia.2017.0278

Yang, J.M., Hsu, Y.J.: Wearable devices for real-time health monitoring: electrocardiography and photoplethysmography. J. Biomed. Eng. **25**(4), 123–135 (2010). https://doi.org/10.1016/j.bmme.2010.03.002

Yang, S., Zhu, S., Zhang, Y., Wang, L.: Convolutional neural networks for predicting Alzheimer's disease progression from MRI scans. Neuroinformatics **19**(4), 589–602 (2021). https://doi.org/10.1007/s12021-021-09576-2

Yun, H., Noh, N.I., Lee, E.Y.: Genetic risk scores used in cardiovascular disease prediction models: a systematic review. Rev. Cardiovasc. Med. **23**(1), 8 (2022)

Zhan, Z., Zheng, Y., Xu, L.: Integrating wearable data with electronic health records for personalized health management. J. Biomed. Inform. **119**, 103837 (2021). https://doi.org/10.1016/j.jbi.2021.103837

Zhang, X., Zhang, S., Chen, X.: Calorie estimation using deep convolutional neural networks. IEEE Trans. Neural Netw. Learn. Syst. **31**(5), 1478–1490 (2020). https://doi.org/10.1109/TNNLS.2019.2939387

Zhang, Y., Wang, X., Huang, X., Wu, J.: Ensemble learning methods for medical image analysis: a comprehensive review. IEEE Access **8**, 63514–63525 (2020). https://doi.org/10.1109/ACCESS.2020.2981464

Zhao, Y., Wang, J., Yang, L., Xu, Y.: Heart rate variability analysis using wearable devices for cardiovascular event prediction. IEEE Trans. Biomed. Eng. **66**(12), 3570–3581 (2019). https://doi.org/10.1109/TBME.2019.2933063

Hardware Analysis for Low-Cost Wearable ECG Monitoring and Analysis System

Shashank Rana, Aditya Handur-Kulkarni, Akhil Binu, Shubhangi Gawali[✉], and Neena Goveas

BITS Pilani K. K. Birla Goa Campus, Sancoale, India
{shubhangi,neena}@goa.bits-pilani.ac.in
https://www.bits-pilani.ac.in/goa/

Abstract. The number of people affected by cardiovascular diseases has been rising rapidly. In many of these cases, the condition is diagnosed late and causes damage and even death of the patient. One way to mitigate this and to encourage more people to record their ECG is to have cost-effective heart monitoring systems for the measurement and analysis of Electrocardiograph(ECG) signals. Personal use heart monitoring systems have been available and rely on various measurements, including electro-mechanical and smartphone-based sensor systems. Many of these are costly, suffer from inaccuracies, and are not easy to use individually or with a combination of other measurements. In addition, these devices are sold by manufacturers with proprietary data capture and storage mechanisms on their cloud-based servers, creating a non-ideal situation for patients in terms of data privacy and the non-availability of raw data for analysis. This paper analyzes various hardware design choices for an ECG monitoring system, which can be made using readily available low-cost hardware. Our prototypes use AD-8232 as a signal amplifier and filter, with 3-pin electrodes for capturing the ECG signals. We incorporate various microcontrollers, including Raspberry Pi Pico W, Arduino Uno R3, and ESP 8266. We use both WLAN and Bluetooth to communicate the captured data. The signals are received on an Android application to process, store, analyze, display, and disseminate the data. We analyze our prototypes for performance metrics and compare them. Our Android application can calculate basic ECG parameters like R-R peak intervals and transmit the data to another device if desired.

We captured ECG data from healthy volunteers when the participants were sitting, walking, running, and climbing. We found that our prototype can be used to measure continuous ECG signals successfully. Our experimental results show that Raspberry Pi Pico W with WLAN is the best for capturing and analyzing continuous ECG data.

Keywords: mHealth · ECG · Wearable Tech · IoT · Ambulatory Health Monitoring

1 Introduction

Traditional devices like Holter monitors have provided long-term ECG signal tracking in cardiovascular health monitoring yet face limitations such as restricted battery life and lack of real-time parameter monitoring. Microcomputer advancements have led to innovative devices utilizing wearable sensors and modern communication technologies. Early systems like the Intel 80196 micro-controller-based heart monitoring system focused on notifying users of abnormal heart rates during ECG signal recording [1]. Recent prototypes integrate GSM/GPRS and Bluetooth modules for communication but encounter challenges regarding smartphone integration and cost-effectiveness if expensive components and specialized boards are used [2].

Alongside these developments, "non-contact" ECG monitoring systems have emerged, offering alternatives to traditional electrode-based methods [3,4]. However, these systems show accuracy and usage-related problems compared to wet ECG sensors. Photoplethysmography (PPG) has been proposed as a non-electrode method for obtaining heart metrics. Studies assessing PPG-based devices have explored their accuracy in detecting atrial fibrillation and analyzing heart rate variability (HRV), revealing encouraging findings that underscore their potential for cardiovascular health monitoring [5].

These technologies for measuring ECG will need a matching system to capture and process the data. In this work, we present a cost-effective solution that can effectively perform end-to-end ECG data processing. In Sect. 2, we present the hardware options and choices we made. In Sect. 3, we detail our complete hardware and software system. In Sect. 4 we discuss our results and in Sect. 5 we present our conclusions and future work.

2 Hardware Components Considered

We considered different options for each component needed for a continuous ECG monitoring system. We focused on readily available and low-cost components that have a good ecosystem for software development. The goal was to choose components that gave a satisfactory level of performance for their task.

2.1 Amplification and Filtration AD8232

The AD-8232 integrated circuit serves as an amplifier and filter for ECG signals. Its Instrumentation Amplifier (IA) with a fixed gain of 100 ensures optimal signal amplification with minimal distortion and is best suited for ECG signals [6]. AD8232 applies a high pass filter and eliminates electrode offsets, minimizing motion artifacts and other noises. AD8232 can operate in standby mode, reducing its power consumption when not in use. The cost-effective AD8232 (18 USD) can also detect when the leads are off and signal the micro-controller accordingly.

Alternate design choices include exploring the pre-amplifier present in ESP-32-based microcontrollers. These, however, are hamstrung by low amplification ratio and lack of ECG-specific filters (Fig. 1).

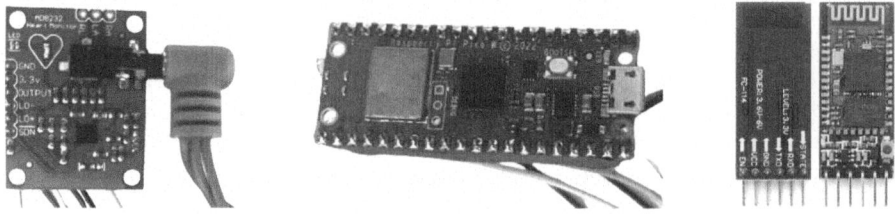

Fig. 1. (a) AD8232 (b) Raspberry Pi Pico W(c) HC-05.

2.2 Micro-controller

Raspberry Pi Pico W. Raspberry Pi Pico W (Pico) board is equipped with a dual-core Arm Cortex M0+ processor and onboard 12-bit Analog-To-Digital (ADC) converter, which serves as the core micro-controller [7]. Pico can read the ECG data through ADC connected to AD-8232. It has an onboard Infineon CYW43439 WiFi module. This module supports 2.4 GHz WiFi (802.11n). Therefore, we can use the Pico to set up a WiFi Access Point. This is the best way to set up a connection, as the IP address of the server on the Pico is fixed. We do not need to change the Pico code, as the client device can connect to it using the IP address. Pico is low cost (10 USD) and is available from many vendors.

Arduino Uno R3. The Arduino UNO R3 (UNO) board is powered by the ATMega328P micro-controller and is equipped with a 10-bit ADC [8], making it good for reading ECG signals but not as effective as the 12-bit ADC supplied with Rpi-pico. Moreover, its limited processing power limits its online signal processing power. By connecting a Bluetooth or GSM module, the Arduino UNO R3 can transmit the ECG data wirelessly to a mobile device. The Arduino UNO R3 is cost-effective (15 USD) and is widely available.

ESP8266. The ESP8266 board, featuring a powerful 32-bit Tensilica L106 processor and a 10-bit ADC, is well-suited for collecting and processing ECG signals from sensors like the AD8232. It can capture ECG data through its ADC and, with its built-in WiFi capability, transmit the data to cloud servers or mobile devices in real-time. This ensures continuous monitoring of ECG signals without the need for additional communication modules. The ESP8266 is both cost-effective (8 USD) and is widely available.

2.3 Communication

WLAN and Bluetooth Classic are the most pervasive communication technologies available on consumer devices. For our use cases, both technologies have a satisfactory range.

Bluetooth Classic HC-05. The HC-05 Bluetooth module operates in the 2.4 GHz ISM band, providing a wireless communication link between the Arduino UNO R3 and other Bluetooth-enabled devices. Supporting Bluetooth Version 2.0+EDR, it offers data rates up to 3 Mbps and a range of up to 10 m, making it sufficient for transmitting ECG data in real-time. The HC-05 is typically interfaced with the Arduino UNO using the hardware serial interface (TX/RX pins). Most devices can connect to multiple Bluetooth devices, allowing users to continue using their other devices, unlike WLAN, which can connect to only one access point.

Wireless Local-Area Network. Wireless Local-Area Network (WLAN) is effective for communication. WiFi for healthcare devices is effective in maintaining data integrity and reducing healthcare costs [9] [10]. We use WiFi operating in the 2.4 GHz band on the Raspberry Pi Pico W and ESP 8266. This provides a robust and high-speed communication method for transmitting ECG data over longer distances than Bluetooth. With data rates of up to 72.2 Mbps (802.11n) and a range of up to 100 m in open space, WiFi enables continuous real-time ECG signal transmission to cloud services or remote monitoring systems using deployed access points or mobile networks. This is superior in terms of bandwidth and range for Bluetooth technology.

3 Proposed System

Our proposed system is a wearable health approach to real-time ECG monitoring in the form of a complete end-to-end pipeline. One of the endpoints is a human connected to an AD-8232 integrated circuit via three electrodes, which can be attached using gell-based stickers. This leads to a microcontroller, which communicates via Bluetooth or WLAN with an Android device running our custom-designed application. This system, as shown in Fig. 2, is cost-effective, lightweight, and portable enough for ambulatory measurements.

3.1 Hardware

From the different options available for hardware and communication, we present results for three different combinations. We chose these as the micro-controller boards have these technologies built on them. Other technologies and boards can also work within our system. The three combinations are:

– UNO with Bluetooth module HC-05
– Pico with WLAN
– ESP82666 with WLAN

These micro-controllers can pull the data from the AD232 board connected to the user. The data received is then sent to an Android application running on a mobile device, as described in Sect. 3.2. The mobile device has to connect to the microcontroller using the WLAN/Bluetooth, depending on the hardware used.

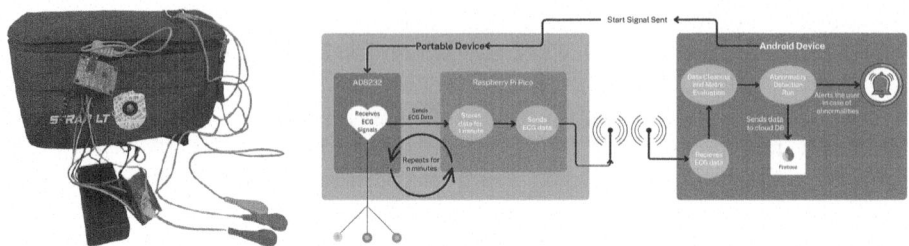

Fig. 2. (Left) Physical setup of the proposed real-time ECG monitoring system showing the wearable components. (Right) Block diagram of the Device and mobile phone components of the system. WLAN or Bluetooth facilitates the communication between them.

3.2 Android Application

We have created a native Android application with Android SDK Level 26 that can execute on more than 95% [11] Android smartphones. Our Android application allows ECG data collection through WLAN or Bluetooth interfaces. The goal of our application is to receive the data, display the data on an interface, and perform an analysis. Mobile devices are becoming powerful enough to detect some abnormalities by running suitable models on them [12]. The features of our application are elaborated in the following sections.

ECG Data Collection. Our Android app is built using the Kotlin programming language. It supports data collection using both WLAN and Bluetooth Classic. In WLAN mode, it establishes a TCP socket connection to the microcontroller; in Bluetooth mode, it discovers, pairs, and connects via a Bluetooth socket to the microcontroller to receive real-time ECG data. The Micro-controller transmits the data packets as a server, while the app functions as the client, receiving and parsing the incoming data using BufferedReader and BufferedWriter Streams. To ensure efficient and responsive performance, asynchronous operations are handled via Kotlin co-routines, enabling background data reception without blocking the user interface.

The data from the server is received and stored locally in the external storage directory. It is then graphically rendered on the application's user interface. We have used GraphView, a custom plotting library for Android, to plot the data. The data stored in the storage can be used for future analysis. This wireless communication method not only eliminates the need for physical connections but also leverages Android's network and storage APIs. This makes our portable, cost-effective, and suitable for real-time ECG monitoring use cases.

Data Cleaning. The ECG signal received from the electrodes attached to the human will contain artifacts corresponding to human breathing, swallowing, etc. These signals are of a different frequency and need to be filtered out. Our application uses the HeartPy library [13] for filtration. The filtered signal is then processed to calculate heart-related metrics like Beats per minute (BPM) and Root Mean Square of Successive Differences between heartbeats (RMSSD). The algorithm used to clean the raw voltage data involves baseline wander removal, a technique most useful for low-frequency noise and drift, often found in physiological signals like ECG. The algorithm uses a high-pass filter to isolate the heart signals from other fluctuations.

Equations for baseline wander removal:

$$Y(t) = X(t) - L(t)$$

Where:

$Y(t)$ is the cleaned signal at time t,

$X(t)$ is the raw signal (voltage data),

$L(t)$ is the low-frequency component representing the baseline wander.

$$\min_b \left(\sum_{i=1}^{N} (x_i - b_i)^2 + \lambda \sum_{i=2}^{N-1} (b_{i-1} - 2b_i + b_{i+1})^2 \right)$$

Where:

x_i is the original signal at point i,

b_i is the estimated baseline at point i,

λ is the regularization parameter,

$\sum_{i=1}^{N} (x_i - b_i)^2$ is the data fitting term,

$\sum_{i=2}^{N-1} (b_{i-1} - 2b_i + b_{i+1})^2$ is the smoothness term.

4 Results

We tested the three hardware combinations as part of our system. These are a Raspberry Pi Pico W transmitting over WiFi, an Arduino Uno R3 paired with Bluetooth classic (via HC-05 module) and ESP8266 with its integrated WiFi module (Table 1). We compared the following parameters: average latency, standard deviation in latency, and overall data quality/error rates. Latency, to a certain extent, can be regulated by adjusting the sampling rate. However, a high sampling rate may overwhelm the microcontroller, resulting in degraded data quality. Given that the size of the QRS complex ranges from 75 ms to 105 ms ([14]), lower sampling rates may lead to inaccurate R-R intervals due to missing the peak.

We experimented with quantifying the overhead for communication in the UNO (copy-to-disk)1. In the copy-to-disk experiment, the Arduino Uno would copy all the data gathered from the AD8232 to its onboard memory. It was later extracted via a USB bridge for further processing.

Table 1. Comparison of sampling delay with added latency for various configurations

Board/System	Sampling delay	Std Dev	Mean
Arduino Uno with Bluetooth	0	11.924	13.228
Arduino Uno with Bluetooth	14	2.6554	13.3574
Copy-to-disk	0	0.8658	12.0621
Pico with TCP	0	18.85	3.49
Pico with TCP	2	1.2169	5.063
Pico with TCP	8	0.62	10
Pico with TCP	14	0.75	16.38
ESP8266 with TCP	2	2.3132	2.1287
ESP8266 with TCP	8	4.0656	8.2610
ESP8266 with TCP	14	4.5107	14.3215

4.1 Arduino Uno with Bluetooth Performance

The Arduino Uno with Bluetooth setup exhibited poor data quality, with instances of dropped/corrupted bits at around a 10-millisecond sampling rate. Although data quality improved at a 14 ms sampling rate, some corrective measures were still necessary at the client end to ensure packet reception. For comparison, we also stored the collected data on the Arduino Uno board's local file system to observe the Bluetooth's impact on transmission. The stored data exhibited no corrupted bits and displayed minimal standard deviation in latency, suggesting that the network limitations of serial communication over Bluetooth Classic cause data corruption.

4.2 ESP 8266 Performance

The ESP8266 board managed lower sampling rates without packet corruption/loss. However, it exhibited a high standard deviation in latency, indicating TCP link instability. This is a problem for time series measurements like ECG, which has a strict requirement for signal processing. A large standard deviation in latency can lead to inaccurate R-R interval estimations.

4.3 Raspberry Pi Pico W Performance

The Raspberry Pi Pico demonstrated low latency for the chosen sampling rate. It showed the lowest standard deviation among all configurations. This is particularly notable for the scenario when no sampling delay was applied. This underscores its suitability for data gathering with strict latency requirements, like what is required for ECG analysis of R-R interval-based calculations of heart metrics and wearable health devices in general.

4.4 Data Capture and User Experience

We captured data using healthy volunteers aged 20–25 years. We collected the data while they were sitting, walking, running, and climbing stairs. The goal was to ensure that our device could be used and gave the required performance in all these kinds of environments. This ensured that our system was robust enough to be used for measurements to obtain health parameters at various levels of activities. Our volunteers could comfortably use our system strapped with a belt and a mobile. We later collected the data that was stored on their mobile device.

5 Conclusions and Future Work

We have presented results obtained from using our system, which ensures end-to-end data collection and complete data privacy. We have implemented a user interface to display the ECG data and analysis done. Future systems could integrate cloud computing for real-time processing of ECG data. This would also enable advanced analytics by leveraging machine learning models.

We also plan to explore alternate design choices, including utilizing higher-end microprocessors for onboard processing and algorithm execution, eliminating the need for a separate smartphone device. This will make our system accessible to people who do not have access or do not wish to use smartphones.

References

1. Alam, M.S., Chatterjee, A., Ferriter, P.: Efficient micro-controller based portable heart monitoring system. In: Proceedings of the 39th Midwest Symposium on Circuits and Systems, Ames, IA, USA, vol. 3, pp. 1264–1267 (1996). https://doi.org/10.1109/MWSCAS.1996.593148.
2. Abidin, Z., Siwindarto, P., Muttaqin, A., Muttaqin, M.A.: Portable heart beat monitoring system using three-lead configuration. Electr. Power Electron. Commun. Controls Inf. Seminar (EECCIS) **2018**, 173–176 (2018). https://doi.org/10.1109/EECCIS.2018.8692840
3. Chen Q., Kastratovic S., Eid M., Ha S.: A non-contact compact portable ECG monitoring system. Electronics **10**(18), 2279 (2021). https://doi.org/10.3390/electronics10182279
4. Silva A., Almeida H., da Silva H., Oliveira A.: Design and evaluation of a novel approach to invisible electrocardiography (ECG) in sanitary facilities using polymeric electrodes. Sci. Rep. 11(1), 6222 (2021). https://doi.org/10.1038/s41598-021-85697-2
5. Jong, G.J., Aripriharta & Horng, G.J.: The PPG physiological signal for heart rate variability analysis. Wireless Pers. Commun. **97**, 5229–5276 (2017). https://doi.org/10.1007/s11277-017-4777-z
6. Analog Devices: Single-lead, heart rate monitor front end data sheet AD8232 (2020). https://www.analog.com/media/en/technical-documentation/data-sheets/ad8232.pdf. Accessed 27 Sep 2024

7. Raspberry Pi Ltd. (n.d.): Raspberry Pi Pico W datasheet. https://datasheets.raspberrypi.com/picow/pico-w-datasheet.pdf. Accessed 27 Sep 2024
8. Arduino S.R.L: Arduino UNO R3 datasheet (2024). https://docs.arduino.cc/resources/datasheets/A000066-datasheet.pdf. Accessed 27 Sep 2024
9. Nagendra, B., Kher, R.: Design and implementation of a low-cost portable ECG monitoring system using a smartphone. IEEE Trans. Biomed. Eng. **66**(3), 756–763 (2019)
10. Pandian, P.S., Muralidharan, R., Rajasekaran, M.P.: Wireless health monitoring system for ECG. J. Med. Syst. **42**(5), 89–93 (2018)
11. Belinski, E., Montiel, F.H.: Android API levels. API Levels (n.d.). https://apilevels.com/. Accessed 27 Sep 2024
12. Shanthi, K.G., Sesha, S., Manikandan, A.: Detection of heart problem using internet of things application. Int. J. Contemp. Res. Rev. **13**, 156–161 (2021)
13. van Paul G., Haneen, F., Nicole, N., Arem, B., Heart rate analysis for human factors: development and validation of an open source toolkit for noisy naturalistic heart rate data (2018). https://repository.tudelft.nl/islandora/object/uuid%3A5c638e14-d249-4116-aa05-2e566cf3df02. Accessed 27 Sep 2024
14. Yanowitz, F.G.: III. Characteristics of the Normal ECG, University of Utah School of Medicine. http://library.med.utah.edu/kw/ecg/ecg_outline/Lesson3/index.html. Accessed 27 Sep 2024

A Method for Detecting Key Fiducial Points in Electrocardiographic Signals for Wave Characterization and HRV Analysis

Luna Panni[1], Gloria Cosoli[1,2(✉)], and Lorenzo Scalise[1]

[1] Dip. Di Ingegneria Industriale E Scienze Matematiche, Università Politecnica Delle Marche, Via Brecce Bianche 12, 60131 Ancona, Italy
`gloria.cosoli@uniecampus.it, g.cosoli@staff.univpm.it`
[2] Dip. Di Scienze Teoriche Ed Applicate, Università eCampus, Via Isimbardi 10, 22060 Novedrate, Italy

Abstract. The analysis of physiological signals is fundamental in fields such as healthcare and sports science, while cardiovascular disease remains a significant global health challenge. This study presents a method for detecting key fiducial points in electrocardiographic (ECG) signals. ECG signals were acquired using the Zephyr BioHarness 3.0 (reference device) and a new wireless ECG device (test device) to conduct the study. Measurements, including wave amplitude and duration, were obtained by identifying these points in the averaged waveform of each ECG signal. Hence, features such as P-wave, QRS complex, T-wave and their relative intervals were extracted from ECG signals provided by both devices. In addition, a heart rate variability (HRV) analysis was conducted, which provides additional information about cardiac health. HRV was analyzed in both time and frequency domains. The results demonstrate the reliability of both devices in identifying significant ECG features, with only minor variations in specific parameters. Notably, the QRS complex shows biases between 0 to 20 ms with percentage differences up to 30%, while the PR interval exhibits biases from 2 to 22 ms and percentage differences up to 33%. The HRV analysis shows strong agreement between the two devices. The study also highlights that both devices consistently measure heart rate (HR) (Pearson's correlation coefficient: 0.88), further validating their accuracy and reliability for clinical and remote monitoring applications. These findings suggest that both devices are suitable for clinical and remote monitoring. Integrating these advanced ECG analysis methods could significantly improve patient monitoring and outcomes in both clinical and non-clinical environments.

Keywords: Metrological Characterization · Electrocardiography · Physiological Data Processing · Heart Rate · Heart Rate Variability

1 Introduction

The importance of physiological signal analysis is increasingly recognized in various fields, including healthcare [1], sports science [2], and wellness monitoring [3]. Cardiovascular disease (CVD) remains one of the leading causes of morbidity and mortality worldwide [4]. The ability to derive information from physiological signals enhances early detection and prevention to reduce the burden of this disease. Moreover, it enables personalized interventions and optimized performance. One of the primary tools for diagnosing cardiovascular conditions is the electrocardiogram (ECG) [5]. Recent advances in wearable and portable technology have improved the ability to monitor and analyze cardiac health through continuous and noninvasive monitoring [6]. These devices, ranging from smartwatches and fitness trackers to specialized medical-grade sensors, have become integral tools for monitoring vital signs such as heart rate (HR) [7], blood pressure (BP) [8], and breathing rate (BR) [9]. By integrating into daily life and providing real-time feedback, wearables enable monitoring outside clinical settings, offering several advantages such as early detection, timely intervention, and the avoidance of ambulatory checks. These advances are crucial in preventing and treating cardiovascular disease, aiming to reduce global incidence and mitigating the related risks.

The morphology of ECG signals reflects the electrical heart activity and conditions [10]. Specific waves characterize each heartbeat, including P-wave, QRS complex, and T-wave. In addition, a small U-wave may be visible in certain ECGs. These waves correspond to different phases of the heart contraction cycle. The P-wave represents the atrial contraction, while the QRS complex and T-wave correspond to the ventricles depolarization and repolarization [11, 12]. Identifying fiducial points associated with these ECG waves is crucial for accurate cardiovascular evaluation, including the diagnosis of arrhythmias [13]. In clinical practice, parameters such as morphology and amplitude of the waves and interval time and segments between fiducial points are essential indicators for ECG diagnosis [14, 15]. Indeed, deviations from typical values can indicate a specific cardiac pathological condition. For instance, the typical ECG values of the P-wave duration, the PR interval, the QRS complex duration, the QT interval, and the T-wave duration are reported in Table 1 [16].

Detecting the QRS complex is the first step when analyzing the ECG signal (e.g., identifying R-peaks and computing the tachogram). Indeed, not only does it provide valuable clinical information, but it can also extract other vital parameters such as HR [14] and analyze its related variability (heart rate variability, HRV) [17]. HRV is a physiological marker that reflects the body ability to adapt to stress and environmental changes [18]. This variability is influenced by the dynamic interaction between the sympathetic and parasympathetic branches of the autonomic nervous system [19].

Table 1. Morphological characteristics in normal ECG [16].

Variable	Duration [ms]	Amplitude [mV]	Remarks
P-wave	80 – 120	0.25	Depolarization of left and right atrium
PR interval	120 – 200	120	Atrial and ventricular depolarization
QRS complex	60 – 120	2.5 – 3.0	Depolarization of ventricles
QT interval	350 – 440	–	Repolarization of ventricles
T-wave	100 – 250	0.1 – 0.5	Ventricular repolarization

In ECG analysis, the R-peak within the QRS complex is the most distinctive and often serves as a reference point for determining other cardiac waves [20]. Various methods have been studied to detect the R-peak and the QRS complex. For sure, the Pan-Tompkins' algorithm [21] is the most classic R-peak detection method. Moreover, Hu et al. [22] introduced an algorithm to detect the onset and offset of the QRS complex. Rabbani et al. [23] introduced a method for detecting R-peaks in ECG signals. They combined wavelet transform (WT), Hilbert transform, and adaptive thresholding. The performance of this method was evaluated against noise and compared with other approaches, showing its superior accuracy in R-peak detection (only this method can accurately detect R-peaks at a noise level of -5 dB). However, detection techniques for identifying fiducial points associated with P and T waves have been explored less. The peaks related to the P and T waves are often identified without accurately determining their start and end points [24]. Kim et al. [25] used a step-by-step baseline alignment approach to detect both the P-wave and T-wave accurately. Madeiro et al. [26] detected the T-wave peak and end [26] using a mathematical model of a skewed Gaussian function. De Palma et al. [27] proposed a thresholding method to detect the QRS complex, P and T waves. Detecting these ECG features is equally important for identifying CVD [28]. Indeed, the precise analysis of the P-wave can provide insights into atrial abnormalities, atrial enlargement, and atrial fibrillation [29]. Similarly, accurately identifying the T-wave can help diagnose conditions like myocardial ischemia, electrolyte imbalance, and other repolarization abnormalities [30]. Changes in the morphology and timing of the P and T waves can indicate ischemia or infarction.

This study has two main objectives:

1. Propose a method for the identification of fiducial points to recognize characteristics waves from ECG signals.
2. Validation of a new wireless ECG device (i.e., test device) with respect to the reference device, Zephyr BioHarness 3.0. Measurements such as wave amplitude and duration are performed by identifying these points in the averaged waveform of each ECG signal.
3. Comprehensive assessment of HRV across the two devices.

The paper is structured into three main sections: Sect. 2 explains the materials and methods proposed, Sect. 3 provides the results, and Sect. 4 discusses these results and draws a conclusion.

2 Materials and Methods

2.1 Acquisition Devices

The ECG signals were acquired simultaneously with two different wearable and wireless devices. The Zephyr BioHarness 3.0 (Zephyr Technology Corporation, Annapolis, MD, US) wearable device [31] monitors physiological parameters, including ECG data. It employs a single-lead ECG configuration by conductive fabric electrodes integrated into the chest strap. This device is FDA-approved and intended for disease diagnosis, treatment, or prevention. It has an accuracy of $\pm$ 1 bpm for the HR measurement, in a measurement range of 0–140 bpm. In this study, it was used as a reference device. The test device is a wireless ECG, referred to as WECG device (Praxe srl). It is designed to capture and transmit physiological data using Bluetooth 5 (Bluetooth Low Energy, BLE) technology. The device receives raw data through a patient cable and communicates this data wirelessly to a receiving computer after establishing a BLE link for data transmission. The WECG device can record 12-lead ECG data by applying 10 electrodes to the patient's body. It directly records leads I, II, and the precordial leads (V1-V6). From these recordings, the remaining leads (III, aVR, aVL, and aVF) can be subsequently derived through mathematical calculations [32], providing a comprehensive 12-lead ECG analysis. It captures additional physiological data, such as acceleration and temperature. The study focuses on WECG signals from the lead II configuration (positive electrode on the left leg, negative electrode on the right arm). Lead II provides a clear representation of heart electrical activity, making it useful for diagnosis.

2.2 Experimental Campaign

The study was conducted at Università Politecnica delle Marche in Ancona, Italy, with approval from the University Research Ethics Committee to comply with the university's Research Integrity Code and the WMA Declaration of Helsinki [33]. The study procedures were explained to the volunteers, who signed an informed consent form. The collected data was handled in compliance with the General Data Protection Regulation (GDPR). Tests were performed on 10 volunteer subjects (21 ± 2 years old, body mass index: 22.1 ± 2.6 kg/m^2 – data are reported as mean $\pm$ standard deviation). The acquisitions from both devices were simultaneous. Figure 1 shows the experimental test setup, including the chest strap placement and the electrodes. Participants were asked to uncover their chest area to allow the placement of the WECG electrodes. They were made to lay on an examination table to ensure they were relaxed and rested. Each acquisition lasted 6.5 min. During the recording, participants were asked to maintain steady breathing and avoid moving to minimize movement artifacts in the ECG signal.

2.3 Data Processing

Feature extraction

The objective was to analyze the ECG data to extract information about P-wave, QRS complex, and T-wave. The data were processed in MATLAB® environment. The signals acquired with both devices were first filtered using the WT to reduce the noise level and isolate the relevant component of ECG. The WT method uses the frequency band division principle [34]. Several mother wavelets were tested, including Symmlet 8, Daubechies 4, Coiflets 4, Bior 3.5, and Haar, and the decomposition level was kept at 6 to adequately cover the ECG frequency spectrum. The signal-to-noise ratio (SNR) and mean square error (MSE) indexes were calculated to find the best mother wavelet, which then was tested across all decomposition levels. With the Pan-Tompkins algorithm, the R-peaks were identified. Each beat was extracted using a temporal window of 250 ms before and 450 ms after each R-peak [35]. Indeed, the R-R interval, which is the interval between the R wave and the next R wave, is between 60 – 120 ms [36]. The 250 ms window before the R-peak is sufficient to include the P-wave and PR segment, which normally last less than 200 ms (Table 1). The 450 ms window after the R peak is sufficient to include the entire QRS complex, ST segment, and T wave. The QRS complex generally lasts less than 120 ms, and the QT interval varies between 350 and 440 ms (Table 1). This ensures that the entire process of ventricular depolarization and repolarization is captured. Since abnormal beats can occur, a further preprocessing step was introduced to discard irregular QRS-complex. In particular, the method described by Varon et al. [37] was applied. The variance of each QRS complex was calculated for accurate identification and classification. Thresholds were set using percentiles and the interquartile range. These thresholds are established based on the 25th (Q1) and 75th (Q3) percentiles, with the interquartile range (IQR) calculated as reported in (1):

$$IQR = Q3 - Q1 \tag{1}$$

A QRS complex was considered irregular and discarded if its variance exceeds the range [Q1 − 2.5·IQR, Q3 + 2.5·IQR]. The average beat waveform was calculated after this preliminary statistical analysis of the beat signals obtained by segmentation. During the parameter detection phase, the analysis of the ECG signals involved several steps. First, the R peak, representing ventricular depolarization, was identified by finding the maximum of the average signal. The other fiducial points were calculated from this index considering the normal ranges reported in Table 1. The Q and S peaks, marking the onset and end of ventricular depolarization, respectively, were determined as local minima in specific time windows of 60 ms before and after the R peak [38], respectively. These windows were chosen based on the typical duration of the QRS complex, which is approximately 60 − 120 ms in a healthy individual. The 60 ms window ensures that the search area encompasses the Q and S peaks while avoiding interference from the P and T waves. Following this, the P peak, representing atrial depolarization, was detected as the local maximum within a window extending from the beginning of the signal to the Q peak. For the T peak, which signifies ventricular repolarization, a window was defined from 100 ms after the S peak to the end of the signal. This choice accounted for cases where a peak with an amplitude greater than 0 mV was observed immediately following the S peak. The 100 ms offset after the S peak is based on the typical duration of the ST segment, which can vary but is usually around 80–120 ms [39]. In the final stage of the analysis, the onset and offset of the P- and T-waves were determined. Initially, windows of 120 ms and 250 ms were created around the peaks of the P- and T-waves, respectively. Then, using the "multithresh" function, the signal values within these windows were divided into nine distinct classes to minimize the variance between the values within each class. Considering Otsu's algorithm [27, 40], the signal was normalized. Finally, the first indices above the threshold were calculated on both sides of the peak. The landmarks obtained as output were used to extract features from the mean beat precisely:

- The P-wave duration was calculated from beginning to end.
- The PR interval from the beginning of the P wave to the start of the Q wave.
- The QRS complex duration from the beginning of the Q wave to the end of the S wave.
- The QRS complex amplitude was calculated as the difference between the mV value of the R peak and the minimum between the Q and S peaks.
- The QT interval from the start of the Q wave to the end of the T wave.
- The T wave duration was calculated from beginning to end.

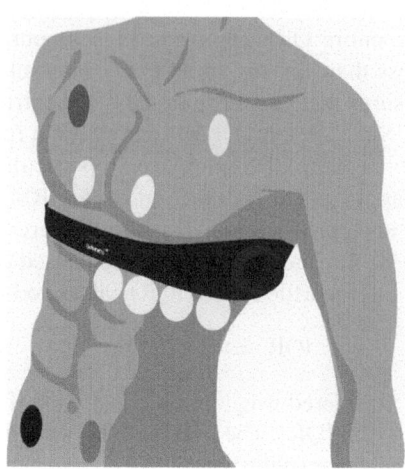

Fig. 1. Experimental test setup showing the placement of electrodes (red: Right Arm, yellow: Left Arm, black: Right Leg, green: Left Leg, white: precordial leads) and the configuration of the WECG device and Zephyr BioHarness 3.0 on a test subject.

Heart Rate Variability Analysis

The HRV analysis was performed in the time and frequency domains. Beginning with identifying R-peaks from the filtered ECG signal, RR interval time series (also referred

Table 2. HRV time and frequency domain metrics.

	Parameter	Units	Meaning
TIME DOMAIN	Mean and std HR	bpm	Variability in HR
	SDNN	ms	Standard deviation of all normal NN interval
	NN50	count	Number of NN intervals differing by more than 50 ms from the preceding interval
	pNN50	%	Percentage of adjacent NN that varied more than 50 ms
	rMSSD	ms	Root Mean Square of successive differences between NN
	HTI	-	Measure the length of NNs on the x-axis and their frequency on the y-axis
	TINN	ms	Triangular interpolation, reference amplitude of the distribution measured as the base of a triangle

(*continued*)

Table 2. (*continued*)

	Parameter	Units	Meaning
FREQUENCY DOMAIN	VLF power	ms2	Absolute power of the very low frequency band [0 – 0.04] Hz
	LF power	ms^2	Absolute power of the low frequency band [0.04 – 0.15] Hz
	HF power	ms^2	Absolute power of the high frequency band [0.15 – 0.40] Hz
	VLF power	%	Relative power of the very low frequency band [0 – 0.04] Hz
	LF power	%	Relative power of the low frequency band [0.04 – 0.15] Hz
	HLF power	%	relative power of the high frequency band [0.15 – 0.40] Hz
	LF norm	nu	LF power in normalize unit
	HF norm	nu	HF power in normalize unit
	LF/HF	-	Ratio of low frequency and high frequency power

to as NN intervals, representing the time between consecutive normal beats) were computed. These RR intervals (i.e., the tachogram) represent the time between successive R-peaks and serve as fundamental HRV analysis data, capturing the HR variability influenced by autonomic nervous system activity. The RR intervals from the ECG signals were used to derive HR values using a sliding window approach for time comparability between the Zephyr BioHarness 3.0 and the WECG data set. In the time domain, analysis focused on the series of NN intervals. The NN intervals can also be transformed into geometric representations [41], including the Triangular Index (HTI) and the NN interval histogram (TINN). The metrics derived are reported in Table 2. HRV measurements in the frequency domain provide insight into the specific contribution of sympathetic and parasympathetic nervous system activities by analyzing the power distribution in different frequency bands. The power of the HRV frequency band was calculated as Welch's periodogram with a Hamming window [42]. The window length was chosen at 10 times the maximum frequency of the signal of interest, and the overlap equal to 50% of the window length to balance spectral resolution and temporal accuracy.

3 Results

This section reports the results of evaluating the extracted features from the average heartbeat waveform and the HRV analysis using the two devices.

3.1 Feature Extraction

Selecting the most suitable wavelet for ECG signal processing, various mother wavelets were evaluated. The Bior3.5 wavelet was found to be the most effective. After testing all its levels, the 1-layer decomposition yielded the highest SNR and the lowest MSE. Therefore, the ECG signals were processed using the Bior3.5 wavelet in 1-level decomposition. The proposed algorithm for detecting key fiducial points for wave characterization was applied to the ECG average waveform signal of 10 different subjects. The landmarks identified by the algorithm were used to extract the features. Figure 2 represents an example of the landmarks identification in Zephyr BioHarness 3.0 and WECG in the average ECG trace of one subject. A statistical analysis was performed for each feature to evaluate the performance and agreement between the WECG device (i.e., test device) and Zephyr BioHarness 3.0 (i.e., reference device). It is essential to understand that the analysis was conducted within the same subject, making it an intra-subject analysis. This means that the extracted features from each device were compared within the same individual to evaluate consistency and accuracy. The calculated metrics include the absolute difference (in ms for time intervals and mV for amplitudes) and percentage difference (%). The results are reported in Table 3.

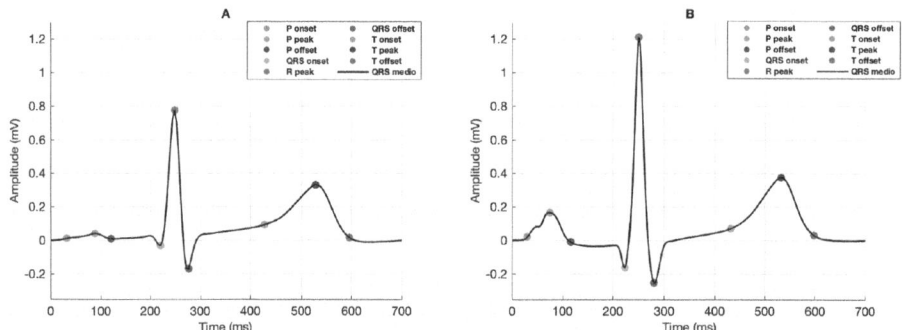

Fig. 2. Example of the landmarks identification in Zephyr BioHarness 3.0 (A) and WECG device (B) in the average ECG trace of one subject. The identified landmarks were then used for feature extraction.

3.2 Heart Rate Variability Analysis

The HRV analysis was conducted in both time and frequency domains. The time domain analysis was applied to the normal inter-beat intervals (NN) series, which were also transformed into geometric representations. The test and the reference device were compared

Table 3. Statistical analysis between Zephyr BioHarness 3.0 and WECG device across 10 subjects indicating bias and percentage differences (%)

Feature	P-wave		PR interval		QRS complex		QRS amplitude		QT interval		T-wave	
Subject	Bias (ms)	%	Bias (ms)	%	Bias (ms)	%	Bias (mV)	%	Bias (ms)	%	Bias (ms)	%
S1	12.00	16.22	2.00	1.27	6.00	9.23	0.40	16.30	0	0	14.00	7.73
S2	6.00	6.90	22.00	13.84	0	0	0.80	32.18	20.00	4.83	0	0
S3	2.00	3.40	6.00	5.60	8.00	14.28	0.66	59.65	2.00	0.54	12.00	7.06
S4	4.00	4.65	8.00	5.90	20.0	30.30	0.12	17.09	14.00	3.80	6.00	3.63
S5	2.00	2.30	6.00	3.14	0	0.00	0.52	43.37	2.00	0.53	2.00	1.20
S6	2.00	2.30	10.0	5.80	4.00	7.41	0.70	47.81	2.00	0.60	6.00	3.82
S7	2.00	2.50	6.00	3.90	6.00	10.53	0.17	9.30	6.00	1.62	6.00	3.40
S8	2.00	2.20	18.00	10.91	12.00	24.00	1.10	48.94	2.00	0.52	6.00	3.31
S9	2.00	2.60	22.00	15.83	4.00	5.40	0.20	8.52	4.00	1.03	10.00	6.13
S10	2.00	2.30	2.00	1.60	8.00	10.53	0.02	1.40	16.00	4.30	14.0	8.30

on a beat-by-beat basis. The performance of the WECG device was evaluated, and the measurement differences (i.e., residuals) with respect to the reference device were analyzed. The distribution of residuals is reported in Fig. 3 for the reference measurement, which was analyzed to derive mean and standard deviation values indicative of the measurement accuracy and precision, respectively. A Gaussian-like distribution is obtained, with a mean value of 0 bpm and a standard deviation of 3.4 bpm. The agreement between the test and reference devices was evaluated through the Bland-Altman plot (Fig. 4). The CI95% of the levels of agreement is equal to [-6.7, 6.5] bpm (coverage factor k = 2) and indicates the measurement statistical confidence. The residuals show no trend with changing HR values, as evidenced by the Bland-Altman plot. Figure 5 illustrates the correlation between the test and reference devices, with a Pearson's correlation coefficient equal to 0.88. In frequency domain analysis, HRV measurements provide a detailed analysis of the power distribution in different frequency bands. A statistical analysis was performed to compare the HRV parameters between the two devices. This comparison focused not on intra-subject consistency but on overall device performance across all subjects. This approach allows for evaluating the devices' reliability and consistency in measuring HRV parameters. The results are reported in Table 4, including mean values, standard deviation for each parameter measured by both devices, and p-value to indicate statistical significance.

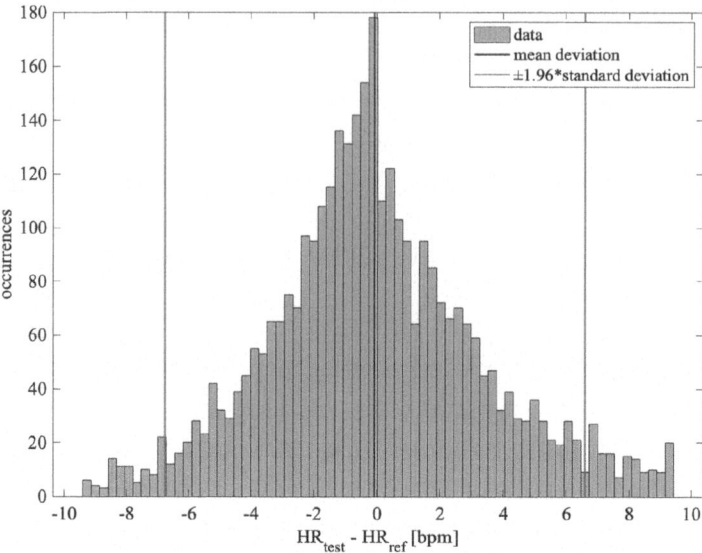

Fig. 3. Distribution of residuals between WECG (test) and Zephyr BioHarness 3.0 (reference) HR measurements. It is possible to observe their Gaussian-like distribution with a mean value of approximately 0 bpm.

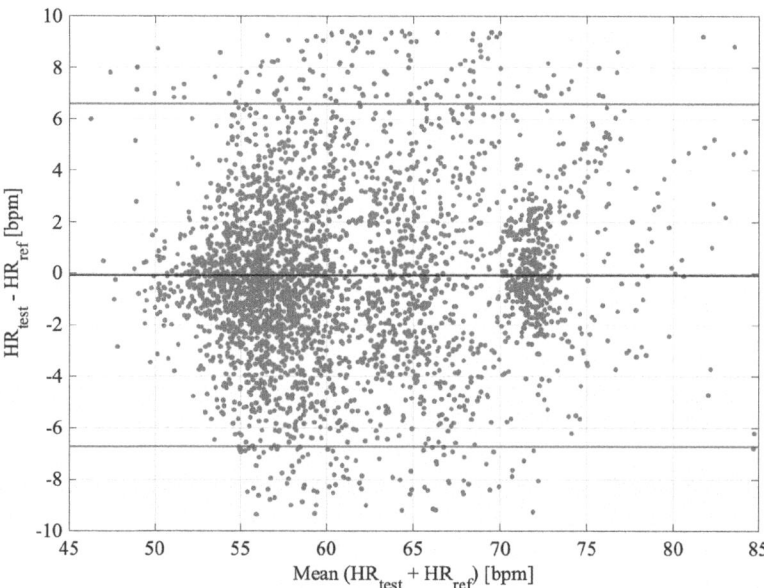

Fig. 4. Bland-Altman plot illustrating the agreement between Zephyr BioHarness 3.0 and WECG. The CI95% levels of agreement are within [-6.7, 6.5] bpm.

A Method for Detecting Key Fiducial Points in Electrocardiographic Signals 127

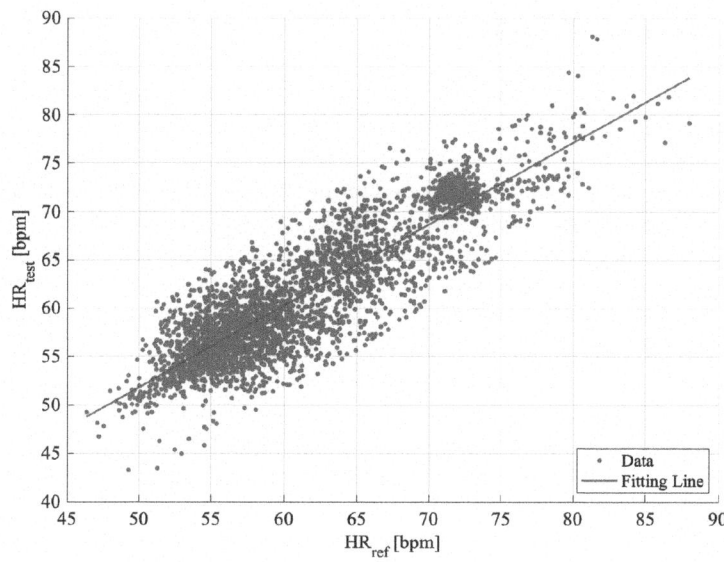

Fig. 5. Correlation between Zephyr BioHarness 3.0 and WECG, with a Pearson's correlation coefficient of 0.88.

Table 4. Comparison of HRV parameters. Mean differences ± SD and p-values indicate the statistical significance of the differences (significance level = 0.05).

Parameter	Mean Difference ± SD	p-value
SDNN	−5.03 ± 10.62	0.17
rMSSD	−6.44 ± 14.27	0.19
NN50	−1.30 ± 8.74	0.65
pNN50	−1.06 ± 2.26	0.17
HTI	0.00 ± 0.50	0.97
TINN	−8.00 ± 21.50	0.27
VLF power	−0.03 ± 0.08	0.30
LF power	−0.27 ± 0.48	0.10
HF power	−0.25 ± 0.42	0.10
VLF power	6.17 ± 11.31	0.12
LF power	−5.88 ± 10.28	0.10
HLF power	−0.53 ± 5.15	0.75
LF norm	−0.10 ± 0.28	0.31
HF norm	−5.03 ± 10.62	0.17
LF/HF	−6.44 ± 14.27	0.19

4 Discussion and Conclusion

The comparative analysis of ECG features extracted from different wearable devices is pivotal in assessing clinical validity, usability, and reliability. In this study, the Zephyr BioHarness 3.0, utilizing a single-lead ECG configuration, was compared with a wireless prototype device, WECG, capable of recording 12-lead ECG data. Lead II from the WECG device was chosen since it clearly represents the heart electrical activity. The study results highlight comparing two ECG devices, Zephyr BioHarness 3.0 and WECG, to extract key ECG features and analyze HRV across 10 test subjects. The extracted features – i.e., P-wave duration, PR interval, QRS complex duration and amplitude, QT interval, and T-wave duration – were subjected to statistical analysis to assess device performance and agreement. Despite the differences in lead configurations between the devices, the results demonstrate that WECG exhibits minimal bias and acceptable percentage differences for most features. For instance, for the P-wave measurements, biases range from 2 to 12 ms with percentage differences mostly under 20%, indicating consistency in measurements. In contrast, the PR interval exhibits biases from 2 to 22 ms and percentage differences up to 33%, suggesting larger variability. The QRS complex shows biases ranging from 0 to 20 ms with percentage differences up to 30%. The QRS amplitude measurements have low biases, up to 1.1 mV. However, the percentage difference reached up to 60%, suggesting significant variability in amplitude measurements between the two devices. This could be attributed to differences in electrode placement. For the QT interval, biases ranged from 0 to 20 ms across subjects, with percentage differences up to 4.8%. T-wave measurements exhibited biases ranging from 0 to 14 ms and percentage differences up to 8.3%. Zephyr BioHarness 3.0 and WECG devices demonstrate variability in their measurements across different cardiac features. Factors such as electrode placement and signal processing algorithm could contribute to these variations. These results underscore the clinical relevance of the measurements obtained from both devices, particularly in diagnosing cardiovascular problems. This study also evaluated HRV measurements obtained from the two ECG devices. HRV is a critical measure in clinical practice, reflecting the autonomic nervous system regulation of the heart. The analysis focused on several key HRV parameters. The results indicate no statistically significant differences between the two devices across these parameters, as evidenced by p-values well above the 0.05 threshold. The time domain metric shows slight mean differences with no significant statistical deviations, indicating that both devices can capture HRV variability. The frequency domain analysis further supports this and demonstrates that test and reference devices provide consistent and reliable HRV measurements. HR measurements were also consistent between the two devices. The close agreement in HR data indicates that both devices can be reliably used for continuous monitoring in clinical settings, everyday scenarios, and sports applications. Moreover, WECG is designed to focus on sports medicine applications, making it particularly valuable during stress testing and physical exertion. Therefore, it can help identify any underlying cardiovascular issues that may only become apparent during physical stress in athletes.

Despite the promising results, this study has limitations. First, the small sample size of 10 subjects may not fully represent the broader population, and further studies with larger cohorts (also in terms of age) are necessary to validate these findings. Second, the study focuses only on lead II for the WECG device, so it does not capture the full potential of its 12-lead configuration. Finally, investigating the impact of environmental factors and physiological states on ECG and HRV metrics will further enhance the utility and reliability of wearable ECG technology in personalized healthcare and sports medicine. Furthermore, incorporating stress tests in future studies can provide a more comprehensive evaluation of the device performance under various physiological conditions. The findings from this study have significant implications for clinical practice, wearable technology development, and sports medicine. Wearable ECG devices offer promising opportunities for continuous monitoring and early detection of cardiovascular abnormalities outside traditional clinical settings. Optimizing algorithms for accurate ECG feature extraction is crucial to enhancing diagnostic reliability and clinical utility. Future research could focus on refining signal processing algorithms, exploring machine learning approaches for automated feature extraction, and validating findings across larger, more diverse patient populations.

References

1. Jeong, J.-W., Lee, W., Kim, Y.-J.: A real-time wearable physiological monitoring system for home-based healthcare applications. Sensors **22**(1), 104 (2021). https://doi.org/10.3390/s22010104
2. Cosoli, G., Antognoli, L., Veroli, V., Scalise, L.: Accuracy and precision of wearable devices for real-time monitoring of swimming athletes. Sensors (Basel) **22**(13), 4726 (2022). https://doi.org/10.3390/s22134726
3. Alhejaili, R., Alomainy, A.: The Use of Wearable Technology in Providing Assistive Solutions for Mental Well-Being. Sensors **23**(17), 7378 (2023). https://doi.org/10.3390/s23177378
4. Di Cesare, M., et al.: The Heart of the World, Glob. Heart **19**, 1 (2024). https://doi.org/10.5334/gh.1288
5. Naples, R., Wang, A., Brady, W.J.: Electrocardiographic tools in clinical care. In: The Electrocardiogram in Emergency and Acute Care, Wiley, pp. 136–142 (2023). https://doi.org/10.1002/9781119266938.ch19
6. Miao, F., Wu, D., Liu, Z., Zhang, R., Tang, M., Li, Y.: Wearable sensing, big data technology for cardiovascular healthcare: current status and future prospective. Chin Med J (Engl) **136**(9), 1015–1025 (2023). https://doi.org/10.1097/CM9.0000000000002117
7. Alugubelli, N., Abuissa, H., Roka, A.: Wearable devices for remote monitoring of heart rate and heart rate variability—what we know and what is coming. Sensors **22**(22), 8903 (2022). https://doi.org/10.3390/s22228903
8. Poli, A., Cosoli, G., Iadarola, G., Spinsante, S., Scalise, L.: Feasibility of blood pressure measurement through wearable devices: analysis of smartwatches performance. In: 2022 IEEE International Symposium on Medical Measurements and Applications (MeMeA), pp. 1–6. IEEE (2022). https://doi.org/10.1109/MeMeA54994.2022.9856533
9. Panni, L., Cosoli, G., Antognoli, L., Scalise, L.: Measurement of respiratory rate with cardiac belt: metrological characterization. Measur. Sens. **34**, 101244 (2024). https://doi.org/10.1016/j.measen.2024.101244
10. deChazal, P., O'Dwyer, M., Reilly, R.B.: automatic classification of heartbeats using ECG morphology and heartbeat interval features. IEEE Trans. Biomed. Eng. **51**(7), 1196–1206 (2004). https://doi.org/10.1109/TBME.2004.827359
11. Aspuru, J., et al.: Segmentation of the ECG signal by means of a linear regression algorithm. Sensors **19**(4), 775 (2019). https://doi.org/10.3390/s19040775

12. McSharry, P.E., Clifford, G.D., Tarassenko, L., Smith, L.A.: A dynamical model for generating synthetic electrocardiogram signals. IEEE Trans. Biomed. Eng. **50**(3), 289–294 (2003). https://doi.org/10.1109/TBME.2003.808805
13. Tsipouras, M.G., Fotiadis, D.I., Sideris, D.: Arrhythmia classification using the RR-interval duration signal. Comput. Cardiol., 485–488. IEEE (2002). https://doi.org/10.1109/CIC.2002.1166815
14. Lee, S., Jeong, Y., Park, D., Yun, B.-J., Park, K.: Efficient fiducial point detection of ECG QRS complex based on polygonal approximation. Sensors **18**(12), 4502 (2018). https://doi.org/10.3390/s18124502
15. Vázquez-Seisdedos, C.R., Neto, J.E., Marañón Reyes, E.J., Klautau, A., Limão de Oliveira, R.C.: New approach for T-wave end detection on electrocardiogram: Performance in noisy conditions. Biomed. Eng. Online **10**(1), 77 (2011). https://doi.org/10.1186/1475-925X-10-77
16. Anbalagan, T., Nath, M.K., Vijayalakshmi, D., Anbalagan, A.: Analysis of various techniques for ECG signal in healthcare, past, present, and future. Biomed. Eng. Adv. **6**, 100089 (2023). https://doi.org/10.1016/j.bea.2023.100089
17. Johnston, B.W., Barrett-Jolley, R., Krige, A., Welters, I.D.: Heart rate variability: measurement and emerging use in critical care medicine. J. Intensive Care Soc. **21**(2), 148–157 (2020). https://doi.org/10.1177/1751143719853744
18. Heiss, S., Vaschillo, B., Vaschillo, E.G., Timko, C.A., Hormes, J.M.: Heart rate variability as a biobehavioral marker of diverse psychopathologies: a review and argument for an 'ideal range.' Neurosci. Biobehav. Rev. **121**, 144–155 (2021). https://doi.org/10.1016/j.neubiorev.2020.12.004
19. Arakaki, X., et al.: The connection between heart rate variability (HRV), neurological health, and cognition: a literature review. Front. Neurosci. **17** (2023). https://doi.org/10.3389/fnins.2023.1055445
20. Sharma, L.D., Sunkaria, R.K.: A robust QRS detection using novel pre-processing techniques and kurtosis based enhanced efficiency. Measurement **87**, 194–204 (2016). https://doi.org/10.1016/j.measurement.2016.03.015
21. Pan, J., Tompkins, W.J.: A real-time QRS detection algorithm. IEEE Trans. Biomed. Eng., **BME-32**(3), 230–236 (1985). https://doi.org/10.1109/TBME.1985.325532
22. Hu, X., Liu, J., Wang, J., Xiao, Z., Yao, J.: Automatic detection of onset and offset of QRS complexes independent of isoelectric segments. Measurement **51**, 53–62 (2014). https://doi.org/10.1016/j.measurement.2014.01.011
23. Rabbani, H., Mahjoob, M.P., Farahabadi, E., Farahabadi, A.: R peak detection in electrocardiogram signal based on an optimal combination of wavelet transform, Hilbert transform, and adaptive thresholding. J. Med. Signals Sens. **1**(2), 91 (2011). https://doi.org/10.4103/2228-7477.95292
24. Li, G., et al.: A new method of detecting the characteristic waves and their onset and end in electrocardiogram signals. Biomed. Signal Process. Control **75**, 103607 (2022). https://doi.org/10.1016/j.bspc.2022.103607
25. Kim, J.-H., Lee, S., Park, K.-H.: P-waves and T-wave detection algorithm in the ECG signals using step-by-step baseline alignment. J. Korea Multimedia Soc. **19**(6), 1034–1042 (2016). https://doi.org/10.9717/kmms.2016.19.6.1034
26. Madeiro, J.P.V., et al.: New approach for T-wave peak detection and T-wave end location in 12-lead paced ECG signals based on a mathematical model. Med. Eng. Phys. **35**(8), 1105–1115 (2013). https://doi.org/10.1016/j.medengphy.2012.11.007
27. De Palma, L., D'Alessandro, V.I., Attivissimo, F., Di Nisio, A., Lanzolla, A.M.L.: ECG wave segmentation algorithm for complete P-QRS-T detection. In: 2023 IEEE International Symposium on Medical Measurements and Applications (MeMeA), pp. 1–6. IEEE (2023). https://doi.org/10.1109/MeMeA57477.2023.10171894

28. Bae, T.W., Kwon, K.K.: ECG PQRST complex detector and heart rate variability analysis using temporal characteristics of fiducial points. Biomed. Signal Process. Control **66**, 102291 (2021). https://doi.org/10.1016/j.bspc.2020.102291
29. Hari, K.J., Nguyen, T.P., Soliman, E.Z.: Relationship between P-wave duration and the risk of atrial fibrillation. Expert Rev. Cardiovasc. Ther. **16**(11), 837–843 (2018). https://doi.org/10.1080/14779072.2018.1533814
30. de Alencar, J.N., de Andrade Matos, V.F., Scheffer, M.K., Felicioni, S.P., De Marchi, M.F.N., Martínez-Sellés, M.: ST segment and T wave abnormalities: a narrative review. J. Electrocardiol. **85**, 7–15 (2024), https://doi.org/10.1016/j.jelectrocard.2024.05.085
31. BioHarness 3.0 User Manual (2012). www.zephyanywhere.com
32. Clinical Electrocardiography: A Simplified Approach. Elsevier (2006). https://doi.org/10.1016/B0-323-04038-1/X5001-X
33. World Medical Association, world medical association declaration of Helsinki. Ethical principles for medical research involving human subjects, Bull World Health Organ., **79**(4), 373–374 (2001)
34. Banerjee, S., Mitra, M.: Application of cross wavelet transform for ECG pattern analysis and classification. IEEE Trans. Instrum. Meas. **63**(2), 326–333 (2014). https://doi.org/10.1109/TIM.2013.2279001
35. Luz, E.J.S., Schwartz, W.R., Cámara-Chávez, G., Menotti, D.: ECG-based heartbeat classification for arrhythmia detection: a survey. Comput. Methods Programs Biomed. **127**, 144–164 (2016). https://doi.org/10.1016/j.cmpb.2015.12.008
36. J. Feher, "The Electrocardiogram," in Quantitative Human Physiology, Elsevier, 2012, pp. 537–546. https://doi.org/10.1016/B978-0-12-800883-6.00050-1
37. Varon, C., et al.: A comparative study of ECG-derived respiration in ambulatory monitoring using the single-lead ECG. Sci. Rep. **10**(1), 5704 (2020). https://doi.org/10.1038/s41598-020-62624-5
38. Riasi, A., Mohebbi, M.: Prediction of ventricular tachycardia using morphological features of ECG signal. In: 2015 The International Symposium on Artificial Intelligence and Signal Processing (AISP), pp. 170–175. IEEE (2015). https://doi.org/10.1109/AISP.2015.7123515
39. Locati, E.T., Bagliani, G., Padeletti, L.: Normal ventricular repolarization and QT interval. Card Electrophysiol. Clin. **9**(3), 487–513 (2017). https://doi.org/10.1016/j.ccep.2017.05.007
40. Otsu, N.: A threshold selection method from Gray-level histograms. IEEE Trans. Syst. Man Cybern. **9**(1), 62–66 (1979). https://doi.org/10.1109/TSMC.1979.4310076
41. Mietus, J.E.: The pNNx files: re-examining a widely used heart rate variability measure. Heart **88**(4), 378–380 (2002). https://doi.org/10.1136/heart.88.4.378
42. Jarrin, D.C., McGrath, J.J., Giovanniello, S., Poirier, P., Lambert, M.: Measurement fidelity of heart rate variability signal processing: the devil is in the details. Int. J. Psychophysiol. **86**(1), 88–97 (2012). https://doi.org/10.1016/j.ijpsycho.2012.07.004

A Minimum Routing Cost Algorithm Based on Quality of Service in Wireless Mesh Networks

Shufan Lin[✉] and Zsehong Tsai

Graduate Institute of Communication Engineering, National Taiwan University, Taipei 10617, Taiwan
{r03942138,ztsai}@ntu.edu.tw

Abstract. Due to the rapid demand of factory expansion, the cost of wired equipment installation is much higher than that of wireless devices. However, wireless network could alleviate much of the costs, so wireless mesh networks (WMNs) play a substantial role in industries now. WMNs enable real-time IP cameras to instantly report on device performance.

We designed an algorithm called Quality of Service (QoS)-Based Centralized Minimum Cost Routing Algorithm (QCMCRA) in WMNs. Before traffic streams flow to its destination, we use a cost function composed of two utility functions to calculate the path cost in WMNs. Additionally, the channel utility function distributes a proper number of channels to each link, restricted by the available number of wireless channels. Finally, we use the proposed delay utility function to check the delay objective of QoS requirement.

The proposed algorithm was evaluated under several scenarios. We used a queue simulator, Java Modelling Tools (JMT), to verify our design comparing to shortest path. By simulation results, we observed that the main advantage of the proposed algorithm is that it satisfies the QoS requirement at a lower path cost than the shortest path. The others are resistance of burstiness and channel fluctuation, load balancing and proper distribution of connections on each link. To sum up, our algorithm achieved desirable outcomes: Finding a minimum cost path within the delay objective of specific QoS.

Keywords: QoS · Delay Objective · Exponentially Bounded Burstiness

1 Introduction

With the proliferation of densely populated areas and smartphones, the prevalence of scenarios with numerous network users and devices is increasing. Our reliance on networks is only growing, with routers connecting devices to the internet and automatically selecting paths. Compared to existing wireless network products, there are many drawbacks to accommodating device access, such as the inability to treat the entire wireless network as a single entity and form a WMN, which limits the benefits of network improvements. In industrial-grade WMNs, router technology and network architecture need to be fully integrated to meet the demands of industrial networks. Furthermore, in this environment, the commonly set QoS targets are statistical delay targets rather than absolute maximum delay times, making the statistics different from those of general mesh networks.

In industrial mesh network application scenarios, factory wireless networks are the most common. As the cost of laying wired equipment increases during factory expansion, wireless devices are becoming more widely used. The demand for devices to connect to the network wirelessly is therefore increasing, leading to increased requirements for wireless networks in industrial settings. Consequently, WMNs have emerged to meet these demands.

WMNs feature multi-hop transmission, self-organization, and self-healing network structures, where numerous routers combine to form a mesh network. Compared to traditional non-mesh networks, they offer higher reliability, adaptability to changes in network topology, and optimization of the overall network. In recent years, research has focused on centralized routing algorithms for WMNs, emphasizing the aggregation of information from each router to a root node, which then calculates the optimal route for all paths by weighting the costs of network paths. This results in a globally optimal route for the entire network, improving routing costs and time delays compared to traditional routing mechanisms.

In industrial environments, equipment developed for industrial-grade WMNs has requirements for QoS, including delay thresholds, total number of wireless channel uses, and wireless channel interference. For example, a traffic flow with 99% of its packets arriving at the destination in less than 200ms is considered to have statistical delay characteristics.

With advancements in technology, router transmission interfaces can now use multiple sending and receiving interfaces simultaneously, and sending and receiving ends can transmit data at different frequencies. While multiple channels can be allocated, issues arise from the simultaneous transmission and reception of multiple interfaces, leading to wireless channel interference. Therefore, centralized management of network transmission by multiple routers composing a WMN can effectively plan routing and meet the service quality requirements of industrial-grade WMNs.

2 Related Work

The research covered in this paper is divided into four main categories: WMNs, routing methods, stochastic queueing models, and utility functions.

The demand for wireless networks has also increased, leading to the emergence of WMNs specifically designed to meet this demand. WMNs feature multi-hop transmission, self-organization, and self-healing network structures, combining countless routers into a mesh network. Compared to traditional non-mesh networks, they offer higher reliability, adaptability to changes in network topology, and overall network optimization [1].

WMNs are expected to be key technologies in the next generation of communication, but there are still many challenges to overcome. Akyildiz et al. [2] discussed various issues such as parameter settings for routing, network scalability, reliability, and stability. At that time, MIMO technology was not widely used, so research began on multi-channel and multi-path routing methods. Benyamina [3] provided a comprehensive overview of WMNs, detailing various design forms and network topologies composed of routers in different shapes, such as triangles, squares, or hexagons. The study analyzes the impact of different shapes on network efficiency.

Routing methods are crucial for path selection in WMNs and greatly affect network performance. Yang et al. [4] proposed a routing method based on evaluating different paths according to their numerical values. The equation consists of two variables: expected transmission time and channel switching cost. Shen et al. [5] mentioned allocating paths based on cost functions, using traffic flow and network load as variables in the cost function for network routing strategies. Chen [6] evaluated WMN routing based on factors such as end-to-end delay, using a cost function to minimize overall network end-to-end delay.

Stochastic queueing models are used to describe the approach of traffic streams approaching statistical upper bounds. Lee [7] viewed Exponentially Bounded Burstiness (EBB) and Exponentially Bounded Fluctuation (EBF) as a problem faced by network transmissions and began deriving its mathematical model and analyzing its impact on networks. Hsu et al. [8] applied the EBB model to their algorithms and wireless APs (Access Points), discussing how the violation probability affects the quality of data or image services.

Chan et al. [9] and Ciucu et al. [10] studied the impact of static routing on network switches. Using the EBB model as the source of network data, they simplified cross-path switches into virtual paths to calculate latency bounds between two nodes and determine whether they meet QoS requirements.

Sharma et al. [11] treated network transmissions as queues and explored the properties of EBB in FIFO buffers. Using the EBB mathematical model, they simulated queues simplified from Markov On-Off Processes to M/M/1 queues and M/D/1 queues in the entire network.

Ciucu et al. [12] described stochastic network calculus, which uses statistical methods to analyze network delays and express delay bounds, simplifying networks using the EBB transmission model. Kadhim et al. [13] and Wang et al. [14] highlighted the increasing importance of WMNs in recent years, comparing network performance using statistical mathematical models to calculate network traffic flow and provide specific boundaries to regulate delay and output.

According to Fidler et al. [15], the Chernoff bound can link the EBB model with the moment-generating function, providing an approximate solution.

Utility functions are used to differentiate functions for different categories or applications. Curescu et al. [16] proposed a concept based on latency classification, assigning lower utility values to low latency and higher utility values to high latency. These functions can be used to distinguish different applications or categories based on their latency requirements.

3 Design

3.1 Stochastic Queueing Model

In this paper, the mathematical model proposed in [7] is utilized to simulate the burstiness caused by transient blocking of data and data blocking resulting from wireless channel fluctuation. This model is used to simulate stochastic network traffic flow and its delay thresholds. Due to the WMN studied in this research, it can be converted into the input-output traffic flow and delay distribution through its mathematical model. This enables the investigation of whether specific proportions of data delay thresholds meet the latency targets for specific QoS. The traffic generation model described in the paper is illustrated in the following figure:

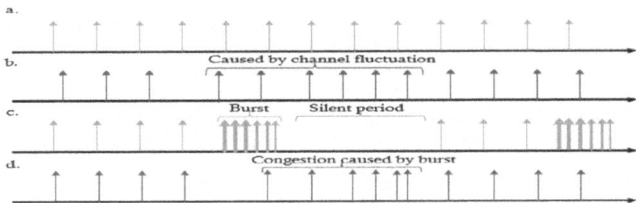

Fig. 1. (a) Initial periodic bit distribution (b) Periodic bits after passing through Wi-Fi EBF channel (c) Initial EBB traffic flow (d) EBB traffic flow after passing through Wi-Fi EBF channel [17].

Random Queue Characteristics. A random process $W(t)$ is said to be Exponentially Bounded (EB) if it satisfies $W(t) \sim (A, \alpha)$:

$$\Pr\{W(t) \geq \sigma\} \leq Ae^{-\alpha\sigma}$$

Traffic Flow Characteristics. A streaming data traffic transmission rate $R(t)$ is said to be EBB if it satisfies $R(t) \sim (\lambda, A, \alpha)$:

$$\Pr\left\{\int_a^b R(t)\,dt \geq \lambda(b-a) + \sigma\right\} \leq Ae^{-\alpha\sigma}$$

Channel Service Capacity Characteristics. The wireless channel capacity $C(t)$ linked to an output node, if it satisfies $C(t) \sim (\mu, B, \beta)$, is termed as EBF:

$$\Pr\left\{\int_a^b C(t)\,dt \geq \mu(b-a) - \delta\right\} \leq B e^{-\beta\delta}$$

When an EBB traffic flow $R(t)$ enters an EBF wireless channel with infinite buffering capacity $C(t)$ using First Come First Served (FCFS) queuing, if $\lambda < \mu$, the output characteristic $S(t)$ of the traffic flow passing through this queue still possesses the characteristics of an EBB traffic flow:

$$S(t) \sim \left(\lambda, \frac{A+B}{1 - e^{-\xi(\mu-\lambda)}}, \xi\right)$$

where $\xi^{-1} = \alpha^{-1} + \beta^{-1}$

When an EBB traffic flow $R(t)$ enters an EBF wireless channel with infinite buffering capacity $C(t)$ using FCFS queuing, if $\lambda < \mu$, the DB (delay bound), $D(t)$, for the traffic flow passing through this EBF queue is:

$$D(t) \sim \left(\frac{A+B}{1 - e^{-\xi(\mu-\lambda)}}, \xi\mu\right) \qquad (1)$$

When multiple EBB traffic flows $R(t)$ enter an EBF wireless channel with infinite buffering capacity $C(t)$ using FCFS queuing, if $\sum \lambda_i < \mu$, as shown in Fig. 2, the DB $D(t)$ for multiple EBB traffic flows passing through this EBF queue is:

$$D(t) \sim \left(\frac{\sum_{i=1}^k A_i + B}{1 - e^{-\xi(\mu(k) - \sum \lambda_i)}}, \xi(\mu(k) - \sum \lambda_i)\right)$$

where $\xi^{-1} = \sum_{i=1}^k \alpha_i^{-1} + \beta^{-1}$, and the set of all traffic flows is $\{1, \ldots, k\}$.

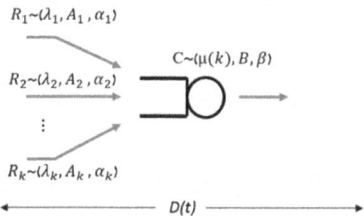

Fig. 2. Multiple EBB traffic flows entering a single EBF queue in the stochastic queueing model [17].

When multiple EBB traffic flows $R(t)$ enter an FCFS queue with infinite buffer capacity $C(t)$ over an EBF wireless channel along their paths, the sum of multiple DBs $D(t)$ along their paths also exhibits exponential bound characteristics, as summed by the following equation:

$$S(t) \sim \left(\sum A_i, \left(\sum \frac{1}{\alpha_i}\right)^{-1}\right)$$

where $R_i(t) \sim (A_i, \alpha_i)$, $i = 1, \ldots, N$.

When multiple EBB traffic flows $R(t)$ aggregate together, the total sum of multiple DBs $D(t)$ along their paths, aggregated using the following formula, also exhibits EBB characteristics:

$$R(t) \sim \left(\sum_{i=1}^{N} \lambda_i, \sum_{i=1}^{N} A_i, \left(\sum_{i=1}^{N} \frac{1}{\alpha_i}\right)^{-1}\right)$$

3.2 Wireless Mesh Network Design

Architecture. In a WMN, all nodes can connect to each other forming a wireless network within the topology. The key difference between a WMN and a typical wireless network architecture is that all nodes can communicate with each other through multiple hops. Multiple parallel wireless channels are allowed between two backbone AP nodes. The graphical representation G using graph theory is defined as follows:

$$G = (V, E)$$

where V represents the set of all nodes v, which can be expressed as:

$$v \in V, \text{where } V = \{v_1, v_2, \ldots, v_i, \ldots, v_j, \ldots, v_{max}\}$$

And E represents the set of all links e, which can be expressed as:

$$e \in E, \text{where } E = \{e_{12}, \ldots, e_{ij}, \ldots, e_{jmax}\}$$

In each link, a certain number of wireless channels need to be allocated, which can be represented as:

$$k \in \kappa, \text{where } \kappa = \{1, 2, 3, \ldots, k_{max}\}$$

where κ represents the set of all available wireless channel numbers k.

Establishing the topology requires understanding the traffic within the network and then allocating wireless channels accordingly. Since the network may initially be in an unused state with no traffic, an initial traffic allocation is calculated before actual transmission. This initial traffic is distributed using the traffic distribution ratio q_{ij}, which is used to allocate the wireless channel numbers based on traffic. By continuously adjusting the traffic size and the allocation of wireless channels, the entire WMN can achieve balance. q_{ij} is defined as follows:

$$\sum_j q_{ij} = 1, \quad \forall i, \quad 0 \leq q_{ij} \leq 1$$

Wireless Mesh Network Model. In the WMN, traffic flows, traffic flow paths, and wireless channels are defined as mathematical models to comply with the methodology proposed in this study.

In a WMN, utilizing 802.11ac with a 20MHz bandwidth in the 5GHz frequency band, 8×8 MU-MIMO (Multi-user Multiple-Input and Multiple-Output), 8 spatial streams, and directional antenna technology. With a 20MHz bandwidth, enough wireless channels are retained for the exclusive use of the WMN while providing an adequate number of available wireless channels to terminals. Therefore, assuming that the remaining wireless channels, excluding those used by the WMN, are available for terminal use, and adjacent nodes in the WMN do not interfere with each other's wireless channels.

When each wireless channel has a bandwidth of 20MHz, if interference occurs in reality, the rate will be adjusted downwards. Under ideal conditions without interference, the theoretical transmission rate can reach 86.7Mbps. The wireless channels in this study are based on a reference value of 86.7Mbps for the theoretical transmission rate, with a maximum achievable transmission rate of 70Mbps for the wireless channels. The transmission rate is fixed and not affected by factors such as interference from wireless channels. By incorporating EBB and EBF designs into the WMN, the transmission delay of transmitted data is increased, resulting in a significant increase in delay for some transmitted data. If the delay of a specific proportion of this transmission exceeds the delay target set for the QoS, it is considered as not meeting the specific QoS; otherwise, it is considered as meeting the specific QoS.

Each flow enters the WMN from a certain node and exits the WMN from another node, with no infinite loop deadlock paths allowed and no loops occurring after splitting. In the process of seeking solutions, the results of infinite loops are eliminated. Each flow can take a single or multiple paths, allowing flows to split after passing through an AP. After passing through an AP, a traffic distribution ratio is assigned to each flow. On each link, the traffic between two nodes is evenly distributed across the active wireless channels k on the link, where k can be less than 3 and greater than or equal to 0. The maximum number of wireless channels k_{max} that can be activated on the same link is three, and the minimum is zero, where no wireless channels are activated on that link. There is no interference between the three wireless channels on the same link. With a 20MHz bandwidth in the 5GHz frequency band under 802.11ac, the total number of available wireless channels is approximately 25. After deducting factors such as interference from radar waves and wireless channels reserved for terminal equipment, the number of wireless channels available for the WMN is approximately 9, denoted as $ch_{max}=9$.

In wireless networking research, symbols like ch_{max} and k_{max} hold significant meanings. ch_{max} indicates the maximum wireless channels available to a single node, while k_{max} represents the upper limit of channels in a link. These symbols are crucial for modeling and analyzing wireless networks efficiently.

Definition of Traffic Flows. In the WMN, there are multiple traffic flows $f_1, f_2, \ldots, f_i, \ldots, f_{max}$. Any traffic flow f_i has its own origin, destination, transmission rate, as well as parameters corresponding to the arrival rate, EBB constant term coefficient, and EBB exponential term coefficient in the queue. The representation of traffic flows is as follows:

$$f \in F, \text{where } F = \{f_1, f_2, \ldots, f_i, \ldots, f_{max}\}$$

Definition of Traffic Flow Paths. Firstly, define the set of paths containing all traffic flows as $p_{m,F}$, where m represents one of the paths in p and F represents all traffic flows $f_1, f_2, \ldots, f_i, \ldots, f_{max}$. The formation of traffic flow paths occurs before any actual transmission, where each node not including the path's endpoint, with the splitting ratio q_{ij}, generates the necessary amount of transmission for computational purposes but no data is actually transmitted. This path is referred to as $p_{m,F}$. When all traffic flows F are contained within the path, it can be abbreviated as p_m. The set of all possible paths for all traffic flows is represented as:

$$p \in P, \text{where } P = \{p_1, p_2, \ldots, p_m, \ldots, p_{max}\}$$

Secondly, define the path of a specific traffic flow f_i as p_{m,f_i}, which only contains the paths traversed by f_i, along with the transmission volumes of all traffic flows F passing through path f_i. This path is denoted as p_{m,f_i}. Expanding the concept in the above equation to individual traffic flow paths, all possible paths for traffic flow f_i are represented as:

$$p \in P, \text{where } P = \{p_{1,f_1}, p_{1,f_2}, \ldots, p_{2,f_1}, p_{2,f_2}, \ldots, p_{m,f_1}, p_{m,f_2}, \ldots, p_{max,f_{max}}\}$$

The detailed data for traffic flow paths includes information such as the path names, their starting and ending points, as well as the load and quantity of unit wireless channels along the link. Each path, denoted as p_{1,f_1}, p_{2,f_1}, ..., p_{m,f_1}, p_{m,f_2}, ..., $p_{max,f_{max}}$, corresponds to specific start and end points, with associated wireless channel loads represented as b_{ab,k_1}, b_{cd,k_1}, ..., b_{ij,k_1}, b_{st,k_1}, ..., b_{xy,k_1}, and quantities denoted as $k_1, k_2, \ldots, k_{max}$. The symbol $b_{ij,k}$ signifies the load distribution among k wireless channels on link e_{ij}, measured in percentage. The symbols p_m, $p_{m,F}$, and p_{m,f_i} denote different aspects of traffic flow paths, indicating the composition and transmission volumes of traffic flows along the path.

Definition of Wireless Channels. The detailed data for wireless channels in links includes information such as the link names, the number of wireless channels, their transmission rates, the service rates at the queue, as well as the EBF constant term coefficients and EBF exponential term coefficients. These parameters are listed for each link, denoted by e_{12}, e_{ij}, ..., e_{jmax}, with corresponding quantities represented as $k_1, k_2, \ldots, k_{max}$, transmission rates as $C_1, C_2, \ldots, C_{max}$

in Mbps, service rates at the queue as μ_1, μ_2, ..., μ_{max} in customers per second, EBF constant term coefficients as B_1, B_2, ..., B_{max}, and EBF exponential term coefficients as β_1, β_2, ..., β_{max}.

4 Method

4.1 Problem Statement

Existing evaluation methods for WMN path selection cannot maintain service quality in the presence of burstiness, where data may experience sudden bursts of transmission within a short period, or when wireless channels are fluctuated causing data transmission blockage followed by a sudden burst of transmission. Current routing methods typically treat factors such as delay as constant values in the evaluation process, without considering delay as a statistical distribution. Therefore, they fail to meet the industrial demand for specific service quality delay objectives.

4.2 Centralized Routing Management

This paper proposes a routing method using a WMN as the research environment to meet the needs of industrial WMNs. It adopts centralized routing management and calculates path costs based on utility functions and cost functions. Under the premise of ensuring SLAs (Service Level Agreements), path costs are evaluated using cost functions, and traffic flows that do not meet specific QoS requirements are assigned extremely high utility values using utility functions. Once the cost function yields a very high utility value through this process, the cost of that path increases. With increased routing costs, paths with higher costs are less favored compared to those with lower costs. By calculating the minimum cost route that meets specific QoS requirements using this cost function, the overall network latency can meet industrial-grade service quality, satisfying the latency goals for different traffic flows.

4.3 Definition of Cost Function

The cost function is defined by the available bandwidth of wireless channels, the number of wireless channels on the link, and the delay target. It is used in the WMN to evaluate which transmission paths can effectively utilize wireless channel bandwidth and the number of wireless channels while meeting the delay threshold.

The cost calculated by the cost function in this paper can determine the path combination with the minimum cost for multiple traffic flows from their respective sources to their respective destinations. The goal is to minimize the overall network cost while meeting specific QoS requirements, as shown below:

$$\text{minimize } cost(p) \text{ subject to QoS requirements} \tag{2}$$

Among all traffic flows $f_1, f_2, \ldots, f_{max}$, find the path combination $p_{m,F}$ that minimizes the path cost. For simplification, $p_{m,F}$ is abbreviated as p_m. Let p_{m,f_i} represent the coefficient m of the path p_m that minimizes the cost function among all paths from the source to the destination under the selection of path p_m for traffic flow f_i:

$$\arg\min_{m} cost(p_m) \tag{3}$$

The cost function is composed of two utility functions: the sum of the wireless channel utility functions of the entire network U_1, and the total product of delay utility functions of the paths U_2. Higher utility values indicate higher costs, meaning a tendency to avoid selecting wireless channel quantities and paths with high utility values, as well as paths that exceed the delay target.

$$cost(p_m) = U_1(p_m) \cdot U_2(p_m) \tag{4}$$

4.4 Definition of Utility Function

A utility function divides the parameter under test into multiple intervals or ranges and assigns different utility values to distinguish the utility values of each parameter interval. It defines the utility function for wireless channels and paths, specifying their utility values based on certain criteria.

Definition of Wireless Channel Utility Function. The wireless channel utility function u_1 is defined as the utility function for a unit link's wireless channel. It is also referred to as the wireless channel utility function or simply channel utility function. The channel utility function employed in this paper aims to achieve a load balance effect by evenly distributing the traffic in the link to the opened wireless channels. This reduces the disparity in the load levels of wireless channels within the same link, preventing overcrowding in highly loaded channels and under utilization in low-loaded channels.

$$u_1(x(k)) = \frac{a_1\left(\frac{x}{b_1} + c_1 - d_1(k-1)\right)}{1 + e^{\left(\frac{x}{b_1} + c_1\right)}} + \frac{a_2\left(-\frac{x}{b_2} + c_2 + d_2(k-1)\right)}{1 + e^{-\left(\frac{x}{b_2} + c_2\right)}} \tag{5}$$

In the provided equation, $a_1 = 500$, $b_1 = 9$, $c_1 = 1.3$, and $d_1 = 0.3$ characterize the first term, while $a_2 = 200$, $b_2 = 5$, $c_2 = 21.3$, and $d_2 = 0.5$ describe the second term. These values define the respective contributions and behavior within the equation.

Where $x(k) = \frac{x}{k \cdot C}$, is the ratio of the link traffic to the number of open wireless channels and their individual wireless channel traffic, i.e., the load of a single wireless channel.

For example, as shown in Fig. 3, the horizontal axis represents the load of a single wireless channel on the same link, in percentage. The vertical axis represents the utility value at that load. For instance, 65% on the horizontal axis indicates that all wireless channels on the same link are loaded at 65%. When

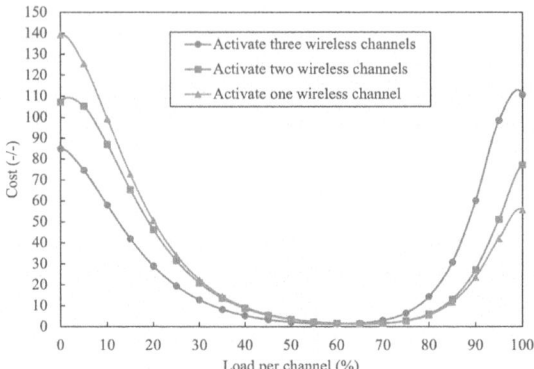

Fig. 3. Curve graph of unit wireless channel utility function load rate against its utility value in the same link.

2 wireless channels are open, the utility value is 1.255. Applying the equation $u_1(x(k))$, it can be represented as $u_1(b_{ij,k})$.

The wireless channel utility function exhibits a U-shaped curve, aiming to encourage movement towards the center of the U-shape for situations concentrated on both sides of the U. These situations include low wireless channel numbers with high loads per channel and high wireless channel numbers with low individual channel loads. Conversely, scenarios with low wireless channel numbers and low channel loads, as well as high wireless channel numbers with high individual channel loads, are less likely to occur after being evaluated by the cost function of paths unless the overall network traffic is very low, the path is the only route available, or the overall network load is excessively high.

The total sum of channel utility function values can be represented as U_1:

$$U_1(p_m) = \sum_{e_{ij} \in p_m} u_1(b_{ij,k}) \tag{6}$$

Definition of Delay Utility Function. Define the delay utility function u_2, setting its utility value in two regions. The purpose is to directly exclude delays that do not meet the required QoS, so a very high utility value is assigned to the portion exceeding the delay target. $D_{max,p_{f_i}}$ represents the individual delay target that traffic flow f_i must meet on its path. If all traffic flows F must meet a specific delay target, it is denoted as D_{max,p_F}, or simply as D_{max}.

$$u_2\left(D_{.x,p_m,f_i}\right) = \begin{cases} 1, & \text{if } D_{.x,p_m,f_i} \leq D_{\max,p_{f_i}} \\ 10^3, & \text{otherwise} \end{cases} \tag{7}$$

The total product of delay utility function values for paths and all traffic flows can be represented as U_2.

$$U_2(p_m) = \prod_i u_2\left(D_{.x,p_{f_i}}\right) \tag{8}$$

4.5 Centralized Routing Algorithm

In the WMN of this study, a centralized network management routing approach is adopted. The advantage of centralized routing lies in the fact that before actual data transmission, each node proactively uploads its information to upper layers until the root node, allowing the root node to obtain the overall network topology. Subsequently, the root node calculates the optimal routes from each source to destination for individual nodes. This routing approach is then used for actual data transmission. The application of centralized routing is primarily beneficial when the source node knows the destination node but is unaware of the best route for the overall network. In this scenario, each node proactively uploads link state information to the central node. The central node then controls routing using this algorithm, ensuring that each source node is directed to its destination via the globally optimal route.

4.6 Wireless Channel Allocation

It is preferable to select channels with minimal interference during the initial setup of the entire mesh network because maintaining wireless channel allocation for an extended period does not support frequent changes. Interference between nodes in a WMN can lead to collisions and data loss if only the same frequency channels are used for transmission. Therefore, properly allocating different frequency wireless channels for data transmission can increase data throughput and reduce the likelihood of collisions.

Regardless of the choice of wireless channel allocation, there are inherent allocation issues. This design adopts static channel allocation, allocating the required wireless channels for links and maintaining them for a long time. Wireless channels are reassigned only when there are changes in the network topology, while ensuring that the channels also balance the load.

4.7 Algorithm for Calculating Channel Utility Values

The algorithm 1 constitutes the upper part of the main algorithm, establishing a table of traffic flow origins and destinations. Sequentially, except for the destination, it calculates the split ratio for each node and its adjacent nodes' links, each having a split ratio. Utilizing the channel utility function, it computes the utility value of each link, identifying the optimal number of wireless channels for the given traffic volume. It records the number of wireless channels corresponding to this utility value, determines the split ratio of nodes that minimizes the total utility value, records the traffic volume for each link, and checks whether the number of wireless channels allocated to each node exceeds the maximum wireless channel limit, denoted as $ch_{max} = 9$.

Algorithm 1. Algorithm for Calculating Channel Utility Values

1: Initialize split ratio on each node without destination
2: Obtain T.R. per link
3: **loop forever**
4: **if** No infinite loop **then**
5:     Calculate T.R. per channel on link
6: **else**
7:     Drop it
8: **end if**
9:
10: $0 <$ T.R. ≤ 100?
11: **if** T.R. is out of bounds **then**
12:     **if** T.R $== 0$ **then**
13:         Disable unused channels
14:     **else**
15:         Continue from line 1
16:     **end if**
17: **else if** T.R is within bounds **then**
18:     Calculate W.C.U. $u_1(b_{ij,k})$ per link
19: **end if**
20: Obtain W.C.U and the number of channels per link
21: Turn on the number of channels on each link
22: Sum total number of using channels per node
23:
24: $\#ch_v \leq ch_{max}$ for every node?
25: **if** $\#ch_v$ exceeds ch_{max} for any node **then**
26:     Drop it
27: **else**
28:     Sum W.C.U. on every link in path $p_{m,F}$
29:     Obtain $U_1(p_{m,F})$
30:     Save $U_1(p_{m,F})$
31: **end if**
32:
33: Estimate all possible paths?
34: **if** There are more paths to estimate **then**
35:     Continue from line 1
36: **end if**

Algorithm 2. QoS Verification Algorithm

1: Load path of $U_1(p_{m,f_i})$
2: Calculate EB characteristics between EBB sources and EBF channels
3: Obtain output characteristics and DB $D(t)$
4: **while** Not arrived at destination of p_{m,f_i} **do**
5:     Arrive destination of p_{m,f_i}?
6:     **if** Yes **then**
7:         Substitute QoS requirement x into $D(t)$
8:         Obtain $D_{.x,p_{f_i}}$
9:         **if** $D_{.x,p_{f_i}} \leq D_{\max,p_{f_i}}$ **then**
10:             Assign $u_2(D_{.x,p_{f_i}}) = 1$
11:         **else**
12:             Assign $u_2(D_{.x,p_{f_i}}) = 10^3$, and drop it
13:         **end if**
14:         Estimate another path of flow f_i
15:
16:         Estimate the paths for all f_i in $p_{m,F}$?
17:         **if** Not **then**
18:             Return to line 1
19:         **else**
20:             Calculate $\prod_i u_2\left(D_{.x,p_{f_i}}\right)$
21:             Obtain $U_2(p_{m,F})$
22:             Load $U_1(p_{m,F})$ of the path
23:             Calculate $cost(p_m) = U_1(p_m) \cdot U_2(p_m)$
24:
25:             Estimate all possible paths in P?
26:             **if** Not **then**
27:                 Return to line 1
28:             **else**
29:                 **if** Exists p_m in P **then**
30:                     Find p_m minimizing $cost(p_m)$
31:                 **else**
32:                     No solution
33:                 **end if**
34:             **end if**
35:         **end if**
36:     **end if**
37: **end while**

The symbols used to compute the utility of a path convey the following meanings: $T.R.$ represents the transmission rates allocated to the links, while $W.C.U.$ denotes the utility of the wireless channel. $\#ch_v$ signifies the total number of wireless channels connected to a node.

4.8 QoS Verification Algorithm

The Algorithm 2 constitutes the latter part of the main algorithm. Using the delay utility function, check if the path meets the delay target set by the QoS. Calculate the DB $D(t)$ of the path based on the parameters EBB and EBF. Substitute the QoS requirements into this to obtain a certain proportion of delay, which is then inserted into the delay utility function u_2. If the delay is less than the delay target, then the delay utility function equals 1; otherwise, it equals 1000. Finally, find the path p_m that minimizes the network cost while meeting the QoS requirements.

5 Experiments

In this section, we perform a validation of the correctness using the process diagram outlined in Algorithm 1 and 2. The study employs network simulation software to verify the proposed mechanism. Furthermore, we provide a brief introduction to the simulation software used in this study, outline the simulation parameters, and validate the approach through case studies.

5.1 Simulation Software Parameters

When simulating real-world scenarios using queueing simulation software, it's essential to establish a correspondence between the parameters in the simulation software and those in the real world.

In correspondence between simulation and real-world parameters, in simulation software, the parameters are denoted as follows: Service rate at the queue μ, customer arrival rate to the queue (λ_1, λ_2), all with a value of 1 customers per second. In the real world, parameters are represented as: Wireless channel transmission rate C, Traffic flow transmission rate at terminal equipment (f_1, f_2), all with a value of 1 Mbps.

5.2 Experimental Design

For this research, we will utilize the mesh topology shown in Figs. 4a and 4b as our experimental cases. Table 1 listing the parameters used to simulate the wireless channels in the queue.

In our preliminary experimental setup, we investigated the amalgamation of high-resolution and regular-resolution image monitoring, referred to as the integrated resolution configuration. Within this arrangement, node APs orchestrated data collection from terminals. Notably, v_1 aggregated data from a combination

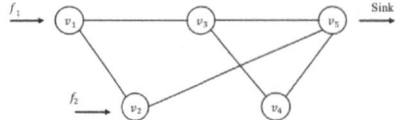 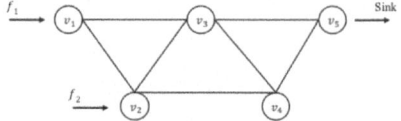

(a) Mesh topology diagrams for experimental cases one and two.

(b) Mesh topology diagrams for experimental cases three and four.

Fig. 4. Mesh topology diagrams for different experimental cases.

of 8k IP Cameras and regular IP Cameras within the integrated resolution setup, while v_2 focused on gathering data from regular IP Cameras. Subsequently, we delved into a configuration exclusively dedicated to regular-resolution image monitoring, termed the Standard Resolution setup. In this context, v_1 monitored regular IP Cameras, while v_2 oversaw regular IP Cameras.

Besides Table 1, in the detailed information of the AP wireless channels, the parameters are as follows: Wireless channel transmission rate C is 70 Mbps, the service rate μ is 70 customers per second, EBB constant term coefficient A is 2.8977, and EBB exponential term coefficient α is 0.7143. Additionally, the EBF constant term coefficient B is 0.0820, and the EBF exponential term coefficient β is 1.6667.

5.3 Measurement of EBB Parameters

To measure the WMNs in this study, it is necessary to first establish traffic flows with EBB characteristics and wireless channels with EBF characteristics. As shown in Fig. 5, the source flow of traffic is a fixed input rate traffic flow that enters the Traffic Generator along with the burst source. The Traffic Generator is a priority FCFS queue. Because the burst source has a higher priority than the source flow, it pushes the source flow to the end of the queue, causing the source flow to line up in the queue. When the burst source finishes serving in the queue, the source flow is released all at once, creating EBB characteristics. After leaving the queue, to maintain the original EBB traffic flow characteristics, the traffic flow generator's exit is set to control the traffic flow rate by branching it to the wireless channel. At this point, the wireless channel has no additional interference from other sources, while the burst source directly flows into the burst sink.

The 1-CDF (Cumulative Distribution Function) of the response time of the traffic source in the wireless channel is measured to find the upper bound of the delay $D(t)$, as shown in Fig. 6. According to [1], when the service rate of the queue is fixed, making $B \to 0$ and $\beta \to \infty$, i.e., EBF $\sim (\mu, 0, \infty)$, the queue does not have stochastic characteristics, and thus, the wireless channel simulated in this study does not have EBF characteristics. Therefore, Eq. 1 can be rewritten as Eq. 9, and by substituting the values, the parameters of the EBB traffic flow, EBB $\sim (\lambda, A, \alpha)$, can be obtained.

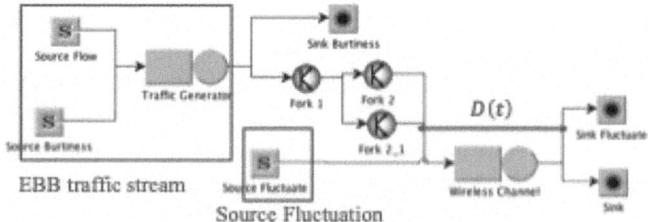

Fig. 5. Model Diagram.

$$D(t) \sim \left(\frac{A}{(1 - e^{-\alpha(\mu-\lambda)})}, \alpha\mu \right), \text{ if } B \to 0 \text{ and } \beta \to \infty \tag{9}$$

where $R(t) \sim (60, 2.8977, 0.7143)$, and $C(t) \sim (70, 0, \infty)$.

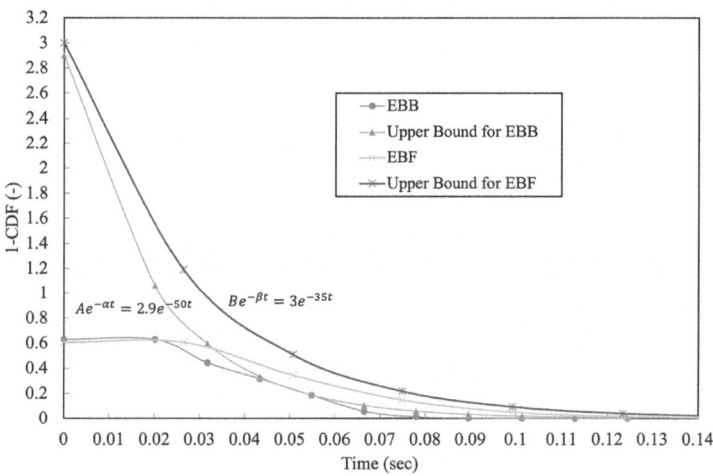

Fig. 6. Upper bound of EBB and EBF.

For the flow priority, λ is 60 Mbps with a service rate of 500 Mbps and a traffic intensity of 0.12. Regarding burstiness, the arrival rate λ is 10 Mbps, with service times $S_{B,peak}$ and $S_{B,non-peak}$ defined by their reciprocal expectations and probabilities. For EBB traffic details, $1/(E[S_{B,peak}]) = 11.11$, interval 1 sec with probability 0.5 (Peak); $1/(E[S_{B,non-peak}]) = 100$, interval 1 sec with probability 0.5 (Non-peak), resulting in traffic intensities of $\rho_{T.G.} = 0.9$ and $\rho_{T.G.} = 0.1$, respectively.

Moving to the wireless channel, we have parameters $\lambda = 60$ Mbps, with a wireless channel service rate of $\mu_{W.C.} = 70$ Mbps, resulting in a traffic intensity of $\rho_{W.C.} = 0.86$. Meanwhile, the priority 3 fluctuate source has a rate of $\lambda =$

20 Mbps, with service times of $1/(E[S_{F,peak}]) = 100$ for peak intervals and $1/(E[S_{F,non-peak}]) = 1000$ for non-peak intervals, leading to traffic intensities of $\rho_{W.C.} = 0.2$ and $\rho_{W.C.} = 0.02$, respectively. Regarding the EBF model details, the service time for peak intervals is $1/(E[S_{F,peak}]) = 100$, with an interval of 1 s and a probability of 0.5, while for non-peak intervals, it is $1/(E[S_{F,non-peak}]) = 1000$, also with an interval of 1 s and a probability of 0.5.

Higher priority numbers indicate higher priority, and vice versa. When the traffic intensity $\rho_{T.G.}$ of the traffic generator is greater than or equal to 1, it causes temporary blocking of the traffic passing through the traffic generator, thereby generating subsequent burst effects. Therefore, the period during which the traffic intensity of the queue is blocked is called the peak.

$$\rho_{T.G.} = \begin{cases} \rho_{T.G.,Flow} + \rho_{T.G.,peak} = 1.02 & \geq 1 \\ \rho_{T.G.,Flow} + \rho_{T.G.,non-peak} = 0.22 & < 1 \end{cases} \quad (10)$$

The average traffic intensity of the queue traffic generator, as given by the following Eq. 11, must be less than 1; otherwise, it will cause continuous blocking of the queue, resulting in the traffic rate entering the queue unable to maintain a constant value upon leaving the queue.

$$\rho_{T.G.,avg} = \rho_{T.G.,Flow} + \frac{1}{2}(\rho_{T.G.,peak} + \rho_{T.G.,non-peak}) = 0.62 \quad (11)$$

5.4 Measurement of EBF Parameters

Traffic flows output from the traffic flow generator have EBB characteristics, and this EBB traffic flow is input into the wireless channel, as shown in Fig. 5. This is because the priority of the fluctuation source is higher than that of the traffic flow source. Similarly, it is analogous to the concept of burst sources and traffic flow sources mentioned earlier. After the fluctuation from this fluctuation source, the wireless channel outputs this EBB traffic flow to the sink, which is the destination. That is, using this queue model to simulate traffic flows with EBB characteristics in WMNs, passing through wireless channels with EBF characteristics.

Measure the 1-CDF of the traffic flow source's response time to the wireless channel and find its upper bound, as shown in Fig. 6. When the service rate of the queue's fluctuation source is not fixed, it can cause fluctuation to the EBB traffic flow passing through. Therefore, by using Eq. 9 to obtain EBB parameters (λ, A, α), and then substituting them into Eq. 1, the EBF parameters (μ, B, β) of the wireless channel can be obtained.

During periods when $\rho_{W.C.}$ exceeds or equals 1, it results in temporary blocking of traffic flows in the wireless channel, leading to fluctuation of EBB traffic passing through the channel, thus endowing the wireless channel with EBF characteristics.

$$\rho_{W.C.} = \begin{cases} \rho_{W.C.,Flow} + \rho_{W.C.,peak} = 1.06 & \geq 1 \\ \rho_{W.C.,Flow} + \rho_{W.C.,non-peak} = 0.88 & < 1 \end{cases} \quad (12)$$

where $R(t) \sim (60, 2.8977, 0.7143)$, and $C(t) \sim (70, 0.0820, 1.6667)$.

The average traffic intensity of the queue wireless channel, likewise, the following equation must be less than 1.

$$\rho_{W.C.,avg} = \rho_{W.C.,Flow} + \frac{1}{2}(\rho_{W.C.,peak} + \rho_{W.C.,non-peak}) = 0.97 \quad (13)$$

5.5 Specific Proportion Delay Estimation

Data is collected using the JMT simulation software to statistically analyze the delay of all data and determine the constant term A_i and exponential term coefficient α_i for the upper bound delay. Based on Eq. 14, the delay $D_{.x,p_{f_i}}$ for a specific proportion x of traffic flow f_i is calculated:

$$x_i = A_i e^{-\alpha_i \cdot D_{.x,p_{f_i}}} \quad (14)$$

After rearranging Eq. 14, the delay $D_{.x,p_{f_i}}$ is obtained as Eq. 15:

$$D_{.x,p_{f_i}} = \frac{\ln A_i - \ln x_i}{\alpha_i} \quad (15)$$

where x_i represents the ratio of traffic flow i not exceeding a specific delay target.

5.6 Software Simulation Diagram

Fig. 7 depicts the implementation diagram in JMT simulation.

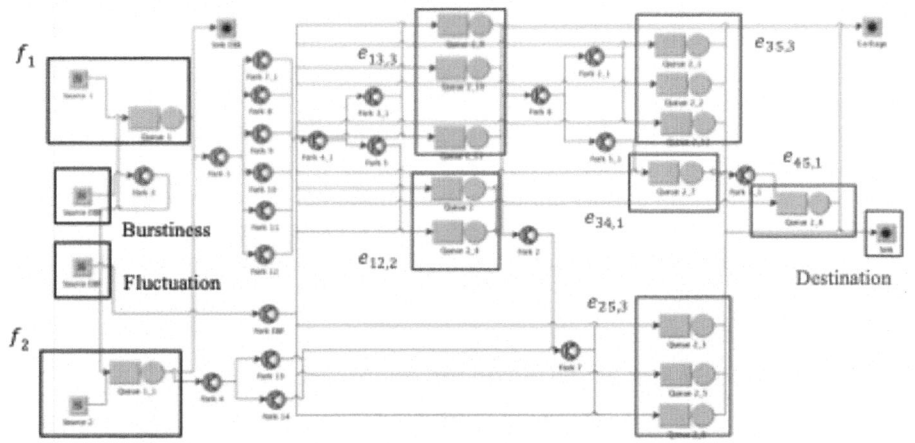

Fig. 7. Software Simulation Diagram.

5.7 Scenario Assumptions

During peak periods of congestion in the queue, the level of fluctuation in the wireless channel is differentiated based on the value of $\rho_{W.C.,peak}$. If $\rho_{W.C.,peak} = 0.2$, it indicates a higher level of fluctuation in the wireless channel, termed as high fluctuation; whereas if $\rho_{W.C.,peak} = 0.1$, it is referred to as low fluctuation.

The experimental group, proposed by this study, maintains the same transmission method regardless of whether the wireless channel experiences high or low fluctuation. The experiment calculates their latency thresholds to compare their resilience to fluctuation in the wireless channel with the control group.

The 802.11ac operates in the 5GHz band with a 20MHz channel bandwidth, allowing for approximately 25 available wireless channels. After accounting for interference from radar signals and channels reserved for terminal devices, the number of usable wireless channels for WMNs is approximately 9, denoted as $ch_{max} = 9$.

5.8 Definition of Control Group

The control group serves as the comparison group for the experimental group. It adopts a shortest path routing strategy, prioritizing entry into a wireless channel in the shortest path link. Only when a certain proportion of the wireless channel capacity is exceeded, another channel in the same link will be opened. For example, when over 90% of the wireless channel capacity is utilized, another channel in the same link will be activated, denoted simply as the control group $\rho_{W.C.,F} = 90\%$.

If all the wireless channels in the shortest path link are already open and the traffic volume has reached 90% of the wireless channel capacity, only then considering diverting traffic to other paths, which also adhere to the aforementioned rules. Once traffic is diverted, it does not return. If after diversion, convergence with other traffic flows exceeds $\rho_{W.C.,F} = 90\%$, the remaining traffic flows are sequentially allocated to the current wireless channel.

The control group employs different transmission strategies depending on whether the wireless channel experiences high or low fluctuation. During low fluctuation, the control group adopts a transmission approach with $\rho_{W.C.,F} = 90\%$; during high fluctuation, the control group adopts a transmission approach with $\rho_{W.C.,F} = 80\%$. This is done to compare its resilience to fluctuation with the experimental group.

5.9 Simulation Scenario Description

The delay targets are established according to the requirements of each traffic flow, where different traffic flows may have different delay targets $D_{max,p_{f_i}}$. After the entire WMN is subjected to varying degrees of channel fluctuation, each wireless channel will have a significant impact on the delay of traffic flows. Therefore, the magnitude of $D_{max,p_{f_i}}$ also needs to be adjusted according to the level of channel fluctuation in the overall WMN. If the fluctuation level is high,

$D_{max,p_{f_i}}$ increases; otherwise, it decreases. If the entire WMN is affected by high channel fluctuation, it will be discussed separately from low fluctuation.

5.10 Results

Referring to Table 2, in the context of high traffic volume, specifically in Scenario 1-1 with high traffic and low wireless channel fluctuation $\rho_{W.C.,peak} = 0.1$, our method effectively distributes traffic across links, achieving load balance and meeting specific QoS latency targets. In contrast, the shortest path method fails to distribute high traffic volumes across multiple links, leading to overloaded individual wireless channels and ultimately failing to meet QoS objectives. Figures 8a and 8b illustrate the scenarios for experimental and control groups, respectively. In Scenario 1-2 with high traffic and overall high wireless channel fluctuation $\rho_{W.C.,peak} = 0.2$, our method demonstrates slight improvement in meeting QoS latency targets compared to the shortest path method, thanks to its load balancing advantages.

Additionally, our method uses slightly more wireless channels but effectively mitigates the impact of high traffic on latency thresholds. Similarly, in the low traffic context, our method outperforms the shortest path method in both low and high wireless channel fluctuation scenarios by maintaining better latency thresholds due to effective traffic distribution and load balancing. Furthermore, our method uses slightly more wireless channels, but the difference is insignificant given the overall network load. In high traffic situations, particularly in Scenario 3-1 with low wireless channel fluctuation, our method excels in load balancing and effectively controls latency thresholds across traffic flows, ensuring adherence to QoS objectives. Conversely, the shortest path method fails to maintain balanced loads, resulting in sharply increased latency thresholds for certain traffic flows and ultimately failing to meet QoS objectives. The use of more wireless channels in our method compared to the shortest path is justified by the need for load balancing under high traffic conditions, ensuring adherence to QoS objectives.

In Scenario 3-2 with high traffic and high wireless channel fluctuation $\rho_{W.C.,peak} = 0.2$, our method continues to effectively distribute traffic and control latency thresholds, while the shortest path method struggles due to its inability to leverage unused wireless channels for effective traffic distribution. Despite using slightly more wireless channels, our method successfully meets QoS objectives by effectively managing traffic distribution. In low traffic scenarios, our method excels in load balancing and latency control, even under high wireless channel fluctuation, ensuring adherence to QoS objectives. Conversely, the shortest path method shows significant increases in latency thresholds, highlighting its inefficiency in traffic distribution and load balancing.

Overall, our method's advantage lies in its ability to balance traffic loads across available wireless channels, ensuring service quality even under challenging conditions, as illustrated across various traffic and fluctuation scenarios.

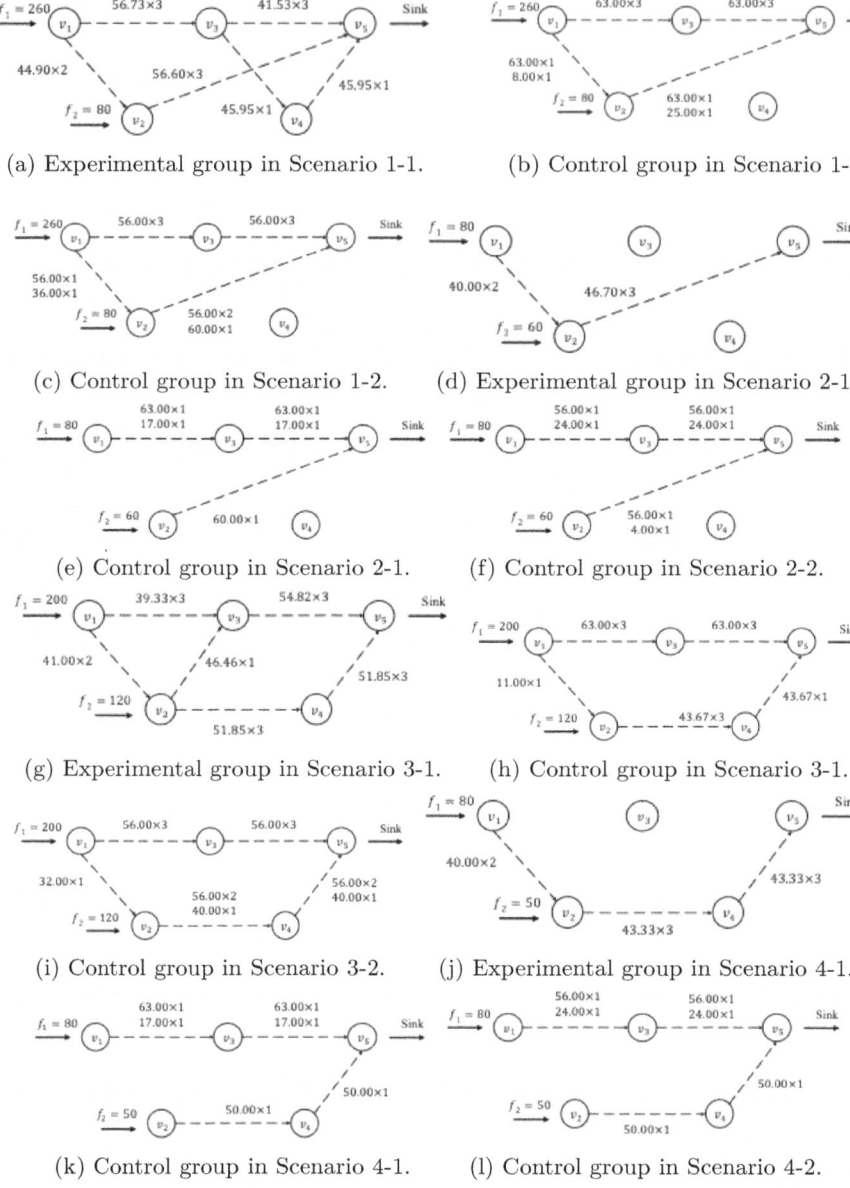

Fig. 8. Comparison of different groups in various scenarios.

Table 1. Traffic flow details. Camera, transmission, regular, and number are abbreviated to cam, trans, reg, and num.

Case	Traffic Flow	Start point	End point	Trans. rate (Mbps)	Arrival rate	Num. of 8k Cams	8k Cam. Traffic (Mbps)	Num. of Reg. Cams	Reg. Cam Traffic (Mbps)
1	f_1	v_1	v_5	260	260	5	250	1	10
	f_2	v_2	v_5	80	80	0	0	8	80
2	f_1	v_1	v_5	80	80	0	0	8	80
	f_2	v_2	v_5	60	60	0	0	6	60
3	f_1	v_1	v_5	200	200	4	200	0	0
	f_2	v_2	v_5	120	120	2	100	2	20
4	f_1	v_1	v_5	80	80	0	0	8	80
	f_2	v_2	v_5	50	50	0	0	5	50

Table 2. Experimental configuration and results

Scenario	Group	Traffic Flow	Wireless Channels	$D_{.95,p_{f_i}}$ (sec)	D_{max,f_i} (sec)	$\rho_{W.C,peak}$	Meets QoS
1-1	Experimental	f1	13	0.2451	0.4	0.1	Yes
		f2	13	0.1984	0.3	0.1	Yes
	Control	f1	11	0.7740	0.4	0.1	No
		f2	11	0.1624	0.3	0.1	Yes
1-2	Experimental	f1	13	0.5767	0.6	0.2	Yes
		f2	13	0.4148	0.5	0.2	Yes
	Control	f1	11	0.6134	0.6	0.2	No
		f2	11	0.5187	0.5	0.2	No
2-1	Experimental	f1	5	0.1635	0.4	0.1	Yes
		f2	5	0.1256	0.3	0.1	Yes
	Control	f1	5	0.4839	0.4	0.1	No
		f2	5	0.1414	0.3	0.1	Yes
2-2	Experimental	f1	5	0.1960	0.6	0.2	Yes
		f2	5	0.1507	0.5	0.2	Yes
	Control	f1	6	0.3803	0.6	0.2	Yes
		f2	6	0.2143	0.5	0.2	Yes
3-1	Experimental	f1	15	0.2603	0.4	0.1	Yes
		f2	15	0.2335	0.3	0.1	Yes
	Control	f1	11	0.7737	0.4	0.1	No
		f2	11	0.1198	0.3	0.1	Yes
3-2	Experimental	f1	15	0.4106	0.5	0.2	Yes
		f2	15	0.3618	0.4	0.2	Yes
	Control	f1	13	0.5514	0.5	0.2	No
		f2	13	0.5015	0.4	0.2	No
4-1	Experimental	f1	8	0.1992	0.4	0.1	Yes
		f2	8	0.1527	0.3	0.1	Yes
	Control	f1	6	0.4743	0.4	0.1	No
		f2	6	0.1228	0.3	0.1	Yes
4-2	Experimental	f1	8	0.2315	0.6	0.2	Yes
		f2	8	0.1782	0.5	0.2	Yes
	Control	f1	6	0.4027	0.6	0.2	Yes
		f2	6	0.1234	0.5	0.2	Yes

6 Conclusion

The algorithm proposed in this study adopts a statistical delay approach to meet specific QoS delay targets in various scenarios, aiming to find the minimum cost routes. Except for extreme cases with high traffic volume and high variability, this method outperforms the shortest path approach. Moreover, the U-shaped utility function proposed in this study has the advantage of (1) load balancing, (2) regulating and closing unused wireless channels, and (3) adapting to wireless channel variability. Additionally, the proposed design can achieve (1) QoS satisfaction and (2) the satisfaction of the maximum available wireless channels for a single node, meeting the high requirements of WMNs.

Simulations were conducted for WMNs, establishing a model with EBB and EBF characteristics. To align with the methodology of this study, traffic flows were defined, traffic flow paths were determined, cost functions were defined to evaluate network-wide costs, and utility functions were defined, comprising wireless channel utility functions and delay utility functions. These utility functions ensure load balancing within the same link and extend to load balancing across the entire network. The delay utility function is used to check if the calculated results meet the research objective of satisfying specific QoS. If the prerequisite is met, the paths that minimize the overall network cost are identified, achieving the research objectives. The proposed methodology is compared with a control group, which prioritizes shortest path routing, regarding the total number of wireless channels, delay thresholds at certain proportions, and QoS satisfaction.

Appendix A: Definitions of Important Symbols

See Table 3.

Table 3. Summary of symbols and their definitions

Symbol	Definition
A_i	Coefficient for the constant term of EBB in traffic flow i
B_i	Coefficient for the constant term of EBF in wireless channel
C_i	Transmission rate of wireless channel, in Mbps
$C(t)$	Time-varying wireless channel capacity
D	Delay time
$D_{\max}$	Delay objective for achieving a specific QoS
$D_{\max, p_F}$	Delay objective of traffic flow F on path p
$D_{\max, p_{f_i}}$	Delay objective of traffic flow f_i on path p
$D_{.x, p_{f_i}}$	$x\%$ delay threshold of traffic flow f_i on path p
$D(t)$	Time-varying delay time of EBB traffic flow through EBF queue

continued

Table 3. continued

Symbol	Definition
G	Directed graph
R_i	Transmission rate of traffic flow i, in Mbps
$R(t)$	Time-varying traffic volume
$U_1(\cdot)$	Sum of utility functions of wireless channels in the entire network
$U_2(\cdot)$	Product of delay utility functions on the path
$\text{cost}(\cdot)$	Cost function
e_{ij}	Directed link from v_i to v_j
f_i	Traffic flow i
k_i	Number of available wireless channels on a single link
$k_{\max}$	Upper limit of the number of available wireless channels on the same link
q_{ij}	Splitting ratio from node i to node j
p	Path
p_m	Path m of traffic flow F, including all traffic volumes on it
$p_{m,F}$	Path m of traffic flow F, including all traffic volumes on it
p_{m,f_i}	Path m of traffic flow f_i, including all traffic volumes on it
$u_1^k(\cdot)$	Unit utility function of wireless channel with k channels
$u_2(\cdot)$	Delay utility function
v_i	Node i
x_i	Proportion of traffic flow i not exceeding a specific delay objective
α_i	Coefficient for the exponential term of EBB in traffic flow i
β_i	Coefficient for the exponential term of EBF in wireless channel
δ	Correction amount for reducing fluctuations
λ_i	Arrival rate of traffic flow i to the queue, in customers/second
μ_i	Service rate of the queue, in served customers/second
$\rho_{W.C.,F}$	Traffic intensity of all traffic flows through the wireless channel
$\rho_{W.C.,\text{peak}}$	Peak traffic intensity of the disturbance source in the queue wireless channel
σ	Burst increase correction amount
ch_v	Number of wireless channels connected to a single node

References

1. Zhang, J., Chai, J., Wang, H., Liu, Y., Yan, B.: Research on centralized self-healing routing algorithm based on wireless mesh network. Electron. Technol. Appl. **41**, 14–17 (2015)
2. Akyildiz, I.F., Wang, X.: A survey on wireless mesh networks. IEEE Commun. Mag. **43**(9), S23–S30 (2005)
3. Benyamina, D., Hafid, A., Gendreau, M.: Wireless mesh networks design-a survey. IEEE Commun. Surv. Tutorials **14**(2), 299–310 (2012)

4. Yang, Y., Wang, J., Kravets, R.: Designing routing metrics for mesh networks. In: IEEE Workshop on Wireless Mesh Networks (WiMesh) (2005)
5. Shen, W., Zeng, Q.A.: Cost-function-based network selection strategy in integrated wireless and mobile networks. IEEE Trans. Veh. Technol. **57**(6), 3778–3788 (2008)
6. Chen, Y.: Mathematical modelling of end-to-end packet delay in multi-hop wireless networks and their applications to QoS provisioning, Ph.D. dissertation, UCL (University College London) (2013)
7. Lee, K.: Performance bounds in communication networks with variable-rate links. In: ACM SIGCOMM Computer Communication Review, vol. 25, no. 4. ACM (1995)
8. Hsu, W., Tsai, Z.: A call admission control algorithm based on stochastic performance bound for wireless networks. In: Advances in Multimedia Information Processing—PCM 2002, pp. 319–328 (2002)
9. Chan, M.C., Lee, T.T.: Statistical performance guarantees in large-scale cross-path packet switch. IEEE/ACM Trans. Network. (TON) **11**(2), 325–337 (2003)
10. Ciucu, F., Burchard, A., Liebeherr, J.: A network service curve approach for the stochastic analysis of networks. ACM SIGMETRICS Performance Evaluation Review, vol. 33, no. 1. ACM (2005)
11. Sharma, P., Bhardwaj, A.K.: Cost function evaluation of routing protocols in wireless mesh networks. Int. J. Comput. Sci. Commun. **3**(2), 280–284 (2012)
12. Ciucu, F., Liebeherr, J.: A case for decomposition of FIFO networks. In: INFOCOM 2009. IEEE (2009)
13. Kadhim, D.J., Jobbar, S.Q., Liu, W., Cheng, W.: The stochastic network calculus methodology. In: Lee, R., Hu, G., Miao, H. (eds) Computer and Information Science, vol. 208, pp. 169–178. Springer, Berlin, Heidelberg (2009). https://doi.org/10.1007/978-3-642-01209-9_16
14. Wang, G., Lai, M., Huang, F., Li, T.: A stochastic network calculus for service performance in wireless mesh networks. In: Computer Science and Education (ICCSE), 2010 5th International Conference on, IEEE (2010)
15. Fidler, M., Rizk, A.: A guide to the stochastic network calculus. IEEE Commun. Surv. Tutorials **17**, 1 (2015)
16. Curescu, C., Nadjm-Tehrani, S.: Time-aware utility-based resource allocation in wireless networks. IEEE Trans. Parallel Distrib. Syst. **16**(7), 624–636 (2005)
17. Yei, C.W.: Providing stochastic delay guarantee in personal area sensor networks. M.S. thesis, Graduate Institute of Communication Engineering (GICE), National Taiwan University, Taiwan, MS (2016)
18. Qualcomm, IEEE802.11ac: The Next Evolution of Wi-Fi Standards, QUALCOMM Incorporated (2012)

Cybersecurity

Navigating Cybersecurity Challenges in Healthcare: Challenges, Innovations, and EU Legal Framework for Connected Medical Devices

Dusko Milojevic(✉) and Maja Nisevic

Centre for IT & IP Law (CiTiP), KU Leuven, Leuven, Belgium
dusko.milojevic@kuleuven.be

Abstract. As healthcare technologies advance, their increasing interconnectivity and integration into more extensive IT networks and systems offer numerous advantages, such as real-time remote monitoring, early prevention and cost reduction. However, this heightened interconnectedness also presents significant challenges, with cyberattacks targeting medical devices and hospital networks emerging as prominent issues. Understandably, the cybersecurity of connected medical devices has gained paramount importance and urgency.

This paper outlines the principal cybersecurity challenges confronting the healthcare sector and introduces insights from the EU-funded CYLCOMED project, which aims to provide the latest technological solutions to address these challenges. Mainly, the paper seeks to identify the primary challenges encountered by the healthcare sector concerning cyber threats. Subsequently, it outlines the high-level architecture of the EU-funded CYLCOMED project (Cyber securitY tooLbox for COnnected MEdical Devices) and its principal objectives, which aim to enhance the cybersecurity of connected, in vitro diagnostic, and software as medical devices (CMDs, IVDs, SaMD). Lastly, it provides a brief overview of the applicable EU legal framework governing the cybersecurity of medical devices.

Keywords: healthcare · cybersecurity · connected medical devices · legal challenges

1 Introduction

The scale and scope of digital transformation in the past decade have been remarkable, leading to significant advancements in everyday life. Previously confined to the domain of science fiction, technologies such as autonomous vehicles, artificial intelligence (AI), surgical robotics, the Internet of Things (IoT), and nanotechnology have become a tangible and integral part of our everyday reality. However, these technological strides, often denoted as part of the fourth industrial revolution (Schwab 2017), have brought about substantial societal challenges, with cybersecurity emerging as one of the most pressing concerns.

The World Economic Forum Global Risks Report (2024) identifies cyberattacks as a substantial global risk. With the increasing reliance on technology in our daily lives, the potential impact and severity of cyber-attacks are growing rapidly. Unsurprisingly, cybersecurity has gained significant traction across the public domain, becoming a top priority on political agendas globally (The White House 2023; Ursula von der Leyen 2021).

In the current cybersecurity landscape, healthcare is one of the most targeted sectors concerning cybersecurity incidents. The European Union Agency for Cybersecurity (ENISA) Report on the health threat landscape (2023a) reveals that the health sector is the third most targeted sector regarding the number of incidents. According to ENISA, patient data, including electronic health records, were ranked as the most targeted assets between January 2021 and March 2023. In addition to the ENISA report, a recent FBI Internet Crime Report (2023) has found that healthcare and public health were the most targeted critical infrastructure sectors in the US in 2023, with 249 officially reported attacks. Successful cyberattacks in healthcare may impede hospital operations, lead to the loss of sensitive patients' data, compromise patient safety, and, in extreme cases, lead to loss of life.

Despite a surge of interest and policy efforts to address cybersecurity challenges, the health sector still lags behind in terms of preparedness and maturity compared to other sectors, such as industrial and financial, to mention just a few.

This article does not seek to provide a comprehensive overview of the complex healthcare cybersecurity landscape. Rather, it concentrates on the foundational background of the proposed CYLCOMED cybersecurity solution. Accordingly, the focus is on something other than presenting real-life case studies or detailed examples of the practical application of the proposed tools and methods. Instead, the CYLCOMED architecture is a central example, offering an entry point to discuss the EU's cybersecurity legal frameworks and the challenges associated with these regulatory structures. The article also does not discuss the weaknesses of existing healthcare hardware devices or compare them with other technological solutions, as its focus is not strictly technical. In line with this course, the article is thereby divided into distinct sections. After a brief introduction, Sect. 2 discusses academic interests in cyberattacks by investigating the security challenges brought about by an increasingly connected medical device and the highly dynamic environment in which it operates. Additionally, Sect. 2 provides precise terminology clarification to facilitate better navigation and understanding throughout this article. Section 3 stresses healthcare cybersecurity challenges by examining connected medical devices. Section 4 provides a brief overview of the CYLCOMED architecture and the main objectives and innovations of the CYLCOMED project, which aims to strengthen the cybersecurity of connected, in vitro diagnostics and software as medical devices. Focusing strongly on the CYLCOMED example, Sect. 5 analyses legal implications by stressing relevant EU legal sources to the cybersecurity of connected medical devices. The last section concludes.

The methodology in this article involves a thematic analysis of existing cybersecurity challenges within the healthcare sector, focusing on Connected Medical Devices (CMDs) and the Internet of Medical Things (IoMT) following the CYLCOMED example. The article reviews critical aspects of the healthcare cybersecurity landscape by referencing recent incidents, challenges and regulatory frameworks. Additionally, the article outlines the structure and objectives of the CYLCOMED project, an EU-funded initiative aimed at addressing CMD cybersecurity. Through a structured examination of EU legal frameworks, including the GDPR, Medical Device Regulation (MDR), NIS2 Directive, and the AI Act, the article stresses the regulatory implications for CMDs' cybersecurity, providing a foundational understanding of how these regulations impact CMD management in healthcare.

2 A Brief Overview of Academic Interests in Cybersecurity of Medical Devices

Over the past five years, there has been a substantial surge in academic interest in cybersecurity in the healthcare sector. A cursory analysis of the Scopus databases highlights this exponential growth, with a notable publication uptick. The analysis, which contained the keywords "Cybersecurity" AND "Health" in their abstracts, has shown that between 2017 and 2023, a total of 724 papers were published (Scopus). This was a clear contrast to the preceding period of 2003 to 2017, during which only 77 papers were published. This surge in research output highlights the increasing recognition of the critical intersection between cybersecurity and health in academic discourse.

Furthermore, the widely cited WannaCry ransomware attack in 2017 is just one of many examples that clearly illustrate the severe consequences of cyber threats in the healthcare sector (Wirth 2017). WannaCry is one of the most intimidating ransomware attacks on health care to this date, which seriously hampered the National Health Service's (NHS) ability to provide patient care, causing the cancellation of nearly 7000 medical appointments, infection of critical medical equipment, and exposure of sensitive patient data, according to National Audit Office Report (2017). It spread to 200,000 machines across more than 100 countries (Walker-Roberts et al. 2018), inflicting a staggering £92 million loss on the NHS (Cyber Security Policy 2018).

In addition to adverse events in 2017, cyberattacks on the IT infrastructure of hospitals, electronic health records, or medical devices during the COVID-19 pandemic have emphasised the critical need to ensure cybersecurity in the healthcare sector (Biasin et al. 2023a). This is clearly exemplified by the Conti ransomware attack on Ireland's Health Service Executive in 2021 (Pattnaik et al. 2023) and the most recent Change Healthcare ransomware cyberattack in 2024, which is labelled as "the most significant and consequential incident of its kind against the US health care system in history" (Pollack 2024, p1).

2.1 Foundational Terms for Navigating Healthcare Cybersecurity

This subsection introduces essential terminology related to connected medical devices to facilitate comprehension of the complex landscape of cybersecurity in healthcare. This makes the article content accessible to a broad audience, including those less familiar with the intricacies of cybersecurity and healthcare technology.

2.1.1 Connected Medical Devices (CMDs)

Once only manufactured to be set up on hospital premises, contemporary medical devices can now generate, collect, analyse, transmit, and store substantial amounts of data while communicating with each other. While the EU Medical Device Regulation (MDR) does not explicitly define the term connected medical devices (CMDs), for clarity in terminology within this paper, *connected medical devices are medical devices that are or incorporate software and artificial intelligence tools, utilising communication technologies, networks, and cloud services to transfer, manage, store, and analyse health data* (Mkwashi & Brass, 2022, p. 9).

2.1.2 Internet of Medical Things (IoMT)

The purpose of enhancing patient healthcare and improving service provision has led to increased integration and connectivity of medical devices into extensive IT systems. Devices like implantable ones (e.g., pacemakers and insulin pumps), wearables (e.g., blood pressure monitors and biosensors), and hospital-based medical equipment are now commonly connected to the Internet, forming what is often referred to as the Internet of Medical Things (IoMT). Notably, the Internet of Medical Things (IoMT) refers to an interconnected ecosystem of medical devices and applications designed to collect, analyse, and transmit health-related data over the internet. Often seen as a healthcare-specific subset of the Internet of Things (IoT), IoMT enables the seamless transfer of patient information, supporting applications such as remote patient monitoring, diagnostic tools, and telemedicine services.

Therefore, the IoMT is an umbrella term encompassing all internet-connected medical devices utilising digital infrastructure for collecting, analysing, and processing health data. However, it is interesting to note that no single and widely adopted definition of IoT exists. It has different meanings to different people. It is sometimes referred to in EU legal acts such as the Data Act (Recital 14) and Cybersecurity Act (Recital 2). However, none of these defines its meaning. The same can be said for the IoMT.

While the Internet of Things (IoT) finds applications in various sectors (Srivastava and Pallavi, 2022), its impact on healthcare is particularly noteworthy, revolutionising the delivery of healthcare services. The IoMT facilitates real-time patient monitoring and behaviour modification, particularly in managing chronic conditions like diabetes and high blood pressure. Its applications in healthcare span from smart hospitals to remote health monitoring, disease diagnosis, and even tracking infectious diseases (Huang et al. 2023).

In the US, for example, there are approximately 10 to 15 internet-connected devices for each hospital bed, and many of these devices are susceptible to cyber-attacks (CISO Global 2018). According to Anderson and Fagerberg (2023), the number of remotely monitored patients reached 56.8 million in 2021. The estimation suggests a compound annual growth rate of 14.2%, anticipating a rise to 126.1 million by 2027.

As connectivity in the healthcare sector has grown, offering benefits like real-time patient care and cost reduction, it has also introduced challenges. The increase in connected medical devices has expanded potential attack surfaces, making each device a potential entry point for cyber threats. With the exponential growth in the number of connected devices, the scale of potential attacks becomes overwhelming. In this complex environment, an attack on one device can compromise the entire system. Scholars, including Yaqoob et al. (2019), have identified seven possible attack vectors within the communication structure of devices interacting with physicians, cloud-assisted data centres, hospital management systems, and data analytics systems. These vectors encompass vulnerabilities in Software/Firmware/Hardware, communication protocols like BLE/ZigBee/Wi-Fi/RF/Ethernet, personal computer or smartphone apps, and app connections to the gateway through Wi-Fi. Exploiting vulnerabilities at multiple entry points can lead to severe consequences.

Next, the foundational concept of the intended purpose plays a pivotal role in the EU regulatory framework outlined by the MDR. MDR Recital 19 offers concise elucidation, specifying instances where software should not be classified as a medical device. Notably, software designed for general or lifestyle purposes, even within healthcare contexts, falls outside the purview of medical devices. However, when a device explicitly articulates a medical purpose, it becomes subject to rigorous MDR requirements. This regulatory paradigm has encountered challenges in the contemporary surge of mobile health applications over the past decade. These applications often emulate functionalities associated with medical devices but, lacking an explicitly designated medical purpose, evade stringent MDR obligations. This exemption raises apprehensions about the adequacy of safety and security standards, particularly concerning user privacy.

The expansion of mobile health applications introduces complexities, making patient data processing less transparent than in conventional healthcare settings. In healthcare scenarios, the revolution of vital patient signs is clearly defined—gathered by sensors, transmitted through communication channels (such as Wi-Fi or Bluetooth) to centralised servers, processed, analysed, and subsequently shared with authorised physicians. Contrarily, in the realm of lifestyle and well-being mobile applications, this data processing becomes obscured, leading to uncertainties regarding data accessibility, potential third-party sharing practices, and the efficacy of safeguarding mechanisms. Unsurprisingly, it is often acknowledged that these apps do not meet even the basic GDPR requirements (Papageorgiou et al. 2018), lack essential privacy safeguards, and lack regulatory oversight (Quinn 2017). Consequently, users of such applications become susceptible targets for cyberattacks.

2.1.3 AI and Cybersecurity

Artificial Intelligence (AI) and Machine Learning (ML) play an increasingly significant role in the cybersecurity of CMDs and IoMT networks. By analyzing patterns in data traffic and device behavior, AI and ML applications can detect and diagnose security threats in real time, providing crucial layers of protection for healthcare systems. These intelligent systems enable the early identification of anomalies and potential threats, continuously adapting to evolving cyber risks, thereby providing essential support for healthcare providers managing connected device security. However, integrating artificial intelligence (AI) applications in healthcare further complicates the challenge of ensuring a secure cybersecurity environment. It is crucial to recognise that complete mitigation of cyber threats is impossible. As expressed by Weber and Studer (2016, p719), the question now is not whether but when a thing such as Medical Health Records (MHR) will be breached. Another underlying challenge is the blurring line between medical devices and mobile health applications (Rak 2021).

2.1.4 The European Union Cybersecurity Legal Frameworks

Cybersecurity legal frameworks are structured guidelines and protocols developed to secure systems, networks, and data against cyber threats. Several key frameworks underpin the European Union (EU) regulatory landscape for cybersecurity in healthcare, such as the EU Cybersecurity Act, Medical Device Regulation, Network and Information System Directive, General Data Protection Regulation, and Artificial Intelligence Act.

3 The Overview of Healthcare Cyber Threat Landscape

According to the EU Cybersecurity Act (2019), cybersecurity encompasses activities to safeguard network and information systems, their users, and others affected by cyber threats. Accordingly, cybersecurity is critical in protecting computer systems and networks from various threats. While delving into the healthcare cybersecurity landscape, it is essential to understand the motivations behind malicious attacks, the associated risks, and the vulnerabilities inherent in the sector.

Malicious cyberattacks can stem from diverse motivations, ranging from thrill-seeking and intellectual property theft to advancing political agendas (Piggin 2017). Furthermore, in cybersecurity literature, financial gain is identified as a primary motivation driving attacks on healthcare infrastructure, given the wealth of sensitive data. Notably, health data holds significant value on the black market, surpassing data from other industries (MacIntyre et al. 2018). In short, Electronic Health Records (EHR) are desirable targets due to their comprehensive nature, encompassing personal information such as birth dates, social security numbers, credit card details, and extensive medical data, including history, diagnoses, medications, radiology images, laboratory results, and mental health conditions. Stolen personal health information can bring substantial sums, ranging from $10 to $1,000 per record, depending on its completeness (Humer and Finkle 2014; Stack 2017). Unauthorised access to such data facilitates additional fraudulent activities, such as submitting false insurance claims (Javaid et al. 2023). Beyond financial motives, ideological reasons and espionage also serve as driving forces for cybercriminals.

A successful cyberattack carries substantial implications with extreme effects on both hospitals and patients. Primarily, security breaches impose additional costs on the healthcare sector, which already operates under financial constraints (Perakslis 2014). According to the ENISA NIS Investments Report (2022), a significant security incident in the health sector has a median cost of 300,000 euros. Besides ENISA, IBM's Cost of a Data Breach Report (2023) identified healthcare breach costs as the highest among industries for 13 consecutive years, increasing by 53.3% since the 2020 report. Hospitals may incur high financial costs due to patient compensation and regulatory fines (Silver et al. 2016). For instance, the Finnish psychotherapy centre Vastaamo faced a fine of EUR 608,000 for GDPR violations related to securing personal data and reporting a data breach (EDPB 2022).

Beyond financial repercussions, the disruption of healthcare services is among the most severe consequences of malicious attacks. For example, during the COVID-19 pandemic, Brno University Hospital in the Czech Republic experienced a ransomware attack, leading to an immediate computer shutdown and the postponement of surgeries (Porter 2020). Similarly, a ransomware attack on a German hospital disrupted emergency services, resulting in a patient's death. While German law enforcement authorities determined that the attack was not directly responsible for the patient's death, such scenarios emphasise the potential for serious harm (Howell 2020). Examples of these incidents significantly damage healthcare reputations, erode credibility, and undermine patient trust (Shenoy and Appel 2017). On a different note, exposing sensitive health data may have harmful effects on patients' well-being, ranging from negative community perceptions to embarrassment, stigmatisation, and even loss of career opportunities (Waegemann 1996).

Alongside violating patient privacy, malicious attacks can lead to physical harm and life-threatening situations. For example, wireless medical devices like insulin pumps and pacemakers can be hacked (Takahashi 2011). Radiofrequency (RF) signals sent to an insulin pump can alter settings and impact insulin dosage, posing potentially fatal outcomes (Levy-Loboda et al. 2022). Due to cybersecurity vulnerabilities in specific insulin pumps, the medical device company Medtronic issued an urgent recall and recommended that patients change to a newer model with enhanced cybersecurity protection (Medtronic 2019).

In achieving all the above-mentioned cyber-attacks, perpetrators employ various malicious techniques, such as ransomware, distributed denial of service (DDoS), hijacking, remote code execution, and social engineering, to achieve their aims. According to ENISA (2023a), ransomware remains the most deployed attack in the health sector in 2023, with an increase in both the EU and globally. ENISA, in the Threat Landscape for Ransomware Attacks Report (2022), defines ransomware as an attack where threat actors take control of a target's assets and demand a ransom in exchange for the return of the assets' availability. Additionally, ENISA (2023b) highlighted the rise of DoS attacks (attacks against availability) in 2023, which are identified as one of the top threats with an upward trend.

3.1 HealthCare Cybersecurity Challenges

The healthcare industry is susceptible to cyberattacks and lags behind other sectors for various reasons. While this article does not delve deeply into these issues, it is crucial to briefly highlight the most pressing ones. Primarily, providing healthcare services has traditionally been oriented towards patient care without considering cybersecurity risks. With the continual evolution of cyber threats, healthcare professionals face additional challenges within an already demanding environment. Notably, the human factor is identified as the most critical element in fortifying cybersecurity in healthcare. Many information security incidents stem from human error, which is consistently acknowledged as the weakest link in the cybersecurity chain (Evans et al. 2018).

The lack of cybersecurity training and awareness among healthcare professionals, combined with a stressful environment, renders them susceptible to attacks rooted in social engineering, such as (spear)phishing and whaling (Al-Qahtani and Cresci 2022).

Besides, the shortage of cybersecurity professionals is well-acknowledged worldwide (ENISA 2020; NIST 2020) and represents one of the biggest challenges in the future (ENISA 2023c). For example, according to the ISC2 (2023) Cybersecurity Workforce Study, the global cybersecurity workforce gap has increased by 26.2% compared to 2021, with 3.4 million more workers needed to secure assets effectively.

The abovementioned challenge is particularly evident in the healthcare sector (Kotz et al. 2016). This is exacerbated by the fact that a medical device cybersecurity expert requires different skill sets than a traditional IT security engineer or architect (Ray Arnab 2021). The Healthcare Information and Management Systems Society's "Healthcare Cybersecurity Survey" (2022) reveals that limited budgets and financial constraints further hinder hospitals' ability to attract and retain cybersecurity professionals. Other underlying vulnerabilities are mirrored in the lack of awareness of cybersecurity issues, training on cybersecurity risks and poor security practices such as password sharing (Williams and Woodward 2015). For example, instances of finding passwords written on notes attached to terminals, sharing access cards, and leaving systems unattended are not uncommon (Yigzaw et al. 2022).

The use of legacy devices is another reason behind the weak cybersecurity posture of healthcare institutions. Medical Device Regulators Forum IMDRF (2023, p8) defines legacy medical devices in the context of cybersecurity as "medical devices that cannot be reasonably protected against current cybersecurity threats". Legacy medical devices in current use were designed and manufactured long before the emergence of cybersecurity threats, therefore, without cybersecurity features in mind. Since medical devices have a long lifespan, many such devices still operate today, using outdated or insecure software, hardware and protocols. For instance, Windows XP is still present in a significant number of today's devices, an operating system with well-known security issues, years after Microsoft formally stopped providing cybersecurity support for it. More worryingly, some hospital equipment is still running on Windows 98, despite Microsoft stopping all support for the operating system in 2006 (Slabodkin 2021). Legacy medical devices have not been manufactured to be connected to the Internet and to communicate with each other, let alone be cyber secure. However, due to financial constraints, the alteration of legacy medical devices with features that facilitate their communication or internet connection is much cheaper than buying new medical equipment. However, these changes to legacy devices are limited since they lack the computational power to perform cryptographic operations without compromising basic functionality and available memory space to accommodate cryptographic software libraries, which makes them a soft target for cybercriminals. Consequently, connecting numerous medical devices and integrating them into large network systems presents a significant challenge, warranting particular attention in the following subsection.

4 CYLCOMED for Cybersecurity of Connected Medical Devices

As cyber-attacks are becoming more intense and sophisticated, the development of robust defensive strategies becomes imperative. A proactive cybersecurity culture is essential, and within this context, the CYLCOMED initiative seeks to fortify the cybersecurity of connected medical devices. The overarching goal is to address the security challenges delineated in this article and elevate cybersecurity standards within healthcare contexts. A primary focus of CYLCOMED lies in enhancing the safety and privacy facets of Connected Medical Devices. The CYLCOMED development of a cybersecurity toolbox follows this objective in supporting comprehensive defence strategies, the architecture of which is provided in Fig. 1.

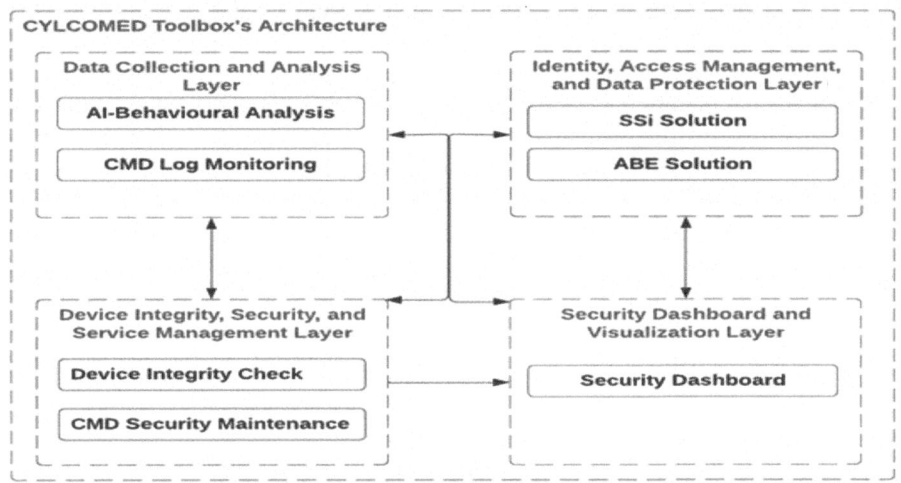

Fig. 1. Current CYLCOMED's Toolbox Architecture

The CYLCOMED toolbox encompasses various tools designed to fortify the cybersecurity of Connected Medical Devices (CMDs). To better describe the structure of CYLCOMED's Toolbox, which showcases modularity, flexibility, adaptability, and efficiency, the tools are organised into four layers forming the final toolbox architecture, as illustrated in Fig. 1.

Data Collection and Analysis Layer collects, monitors, and analyses data from diverse sources within the CYLCOMED ecosystem to detect potential cybersecurity threats or anomalies proactively. It integrates two core components: the CMD Log Monitoring system and the behavioural analysis tool. These tools leverage artificial intelligence to examine logs and network traffic generated by connected medical devices and the platforms managing them. The aim is to identify unusual patterns or activities that could indicate a potential security incident. The primary function of this layer is to provide real-time, continuous surveillance of system activities, ensuring the prompt detection and response to emerging threats. It aggregates and processes large volumes of data from various sources, including network traffic, device logs, and other relevant streams, applying sophisticated algorithms to detect deviations from normal behaviour. This approach enables the system to recognise even subtle signs of potential compromise. By constantly monitoring and analysing these signs, this layer plays a vital role in enhancing the security posture of the CYLCOMED ecosystem, helping to safeguard the integrity and reliability of the connected medical infrastructure. For instance, while AI-based CMD Behavioral Analysis utilises machine learning algorithms to scrutinise data transmission patterns from CMDs and identify abnormalities indicative of security breaches, AI-powered Log Monitoring aims to automatically detect anomalies in system/application logs, thus improving performance and ensuring security.

Device Integrity, Security and Service Management Layer's primary objective is to uphold the operational integrity of medical devices, safeguarding them against unauthorised modifications and ensuring their lifecycle management remains secure. This layer includes mechanisms facilitating secure firmware updates and configurations aligned with healthcare standards and regulations. These protections not only prevent tampering but also ensure that updates and configurations meet strict regulatory requirements, thereby enhancing device reliability and patient safety throughout the device's lifecycle. Tools integrated into this layer serve two main functions. First, they enable connected medical devices' security maintenance by establishing a secure management infrastructure for device updates and configurations, ultimately minimising the attack surface. Second, they provide connected medical device integrity checks, focusing on preserving security features and ensuring the integrity of the devices without compromising their regulatory certification.

Hence, the tools integrated into this layer prioritise essential functionalities to optimise service delivery, strengthen security, and improve operational efficiency, specifically:

- Ensure secure updates of services on medical devices.
- Reduce the attack surface for both medical devices and cloud infrastructure.
- Detect misconfigurations promptly.
- Maintain code integrity and configuration integrity across all connected medical devices.

The identity, Access Management, and Data Protection Layer establishes strong access control and data protection mechanisms tailored to healthcare's unique requirements. This layer enforces encryption and secure data-sharing protocols, acting as the system's gatekeeper by managing access through predefined policies and user roles to uphold data privacy and comply with legal and ethical standards.

Built on a decentralised self-sovereign identity framework, this layer prioritises patient privacy and the confidentiality of sensitive data produced by CMDs, ensuring that unauthorised data access is effectively prevented. Additionally, CYLCOMED's data protection approach, centred on encrypting CMD-generated data, aligns with regulatory requirements, such as the General Data Protection Regulation, and secures data both in transit and at rest, thereby reducing cybersecurity risks. For instance, this layer's Decentralized Identity Management and Data Protection tools enhance identity management and data security through a decentralised approach, enabling privacy-preserving, secure data exchange between devices and healthcare providers. This is achieved using advanced encryption methods, such as Ciphertext-Policy Attribute-Based Encryption (CP-ABE), which facilitates secure, controlled access to data while maintaining patient privacy and confidentiality.

The Security Dashboard and Visualization Layer is the topmost layer of the CYLCOMED architecture. The Security Dashboard provides a comprehensive view of the system's cybersecurity state by centralizing the reporting and visualization of security alerts, anomalies, and metrics. Serving as a centralised Security Information and Event Management (SIEM) tool, its primary function is to aggregate, analyse, and display security data from across the CYLCOMED framework, delivering real-time situational awareness for cybersecurity events and enabling timely and effective incident response.

This dashboard synthesises data from various sources, including the AI Behavioural Analysis component, network traffic monitoring, and vulnerability assessments, to produce a continuous and accurate representation of the security status of connected medical devices. Its key responsibilities within the CYLCOMED framework are:

- Real-time monitoring of connected medical devices,
- Alert generation and incident notification,
- Vulnerability assessment and management to proactively address security risks and
- Comprehensive reporting and analysis to support evidence-based security decision-making.

This layer is integral to sustaining the integrity and security of the CYLCOMED ecosystem, providing the analytical depth required for a resilient cybersecurity posture.

Collectively, these tools contribute to CYLCOMED's mission of enhancing cybersecurity standards and mitigating potential threats in the realm of Connected Medical Devices. The performance and applicability of the CYLCOMED technical solutions will be demonstrated by implementing the developed tools in two dedicated pilots.

Pilot 1 (Fig. 2), Cybersecurity in Hospital Equipment for COVID-19 ICU Patients, will be carried out as a digital twin simulation without direct human participation. This pilot focuses on a muscular relaxation infusion controller, a medical device vital for COVID-19 ICU patients. The controller measures the patient's relaxometry levels, adjusting infusion doses accordingly. The infusion pump is regulated, and alarms manage relaxation levels automatically. The pilot, conducted in a controlled laboratory environment, is a proof of concept with no involvement of actual patients. Critical aspects of Pilot 1 include:

- **Test Scenario**: A prototypical implementation of the testbench and an autonomous intelligent controller assesses the functionality and performance of the muscular relaxation infusion controller.
- **Objective: To** test the connected medical device integrity solution and address the medical equipment needs in an "on-premises" scenario.
- **Interaction with CYLCOMED**: The CMD interacts with CYLCOMED through a single-board computer, emphasising the connected medical device integrity solution as the core, complemented by other tools offering their benefits.

This pilot aims to demonstrate the practicality and effectiveness of CYLCOMED's technical solutions in a simulated healthcare environment.

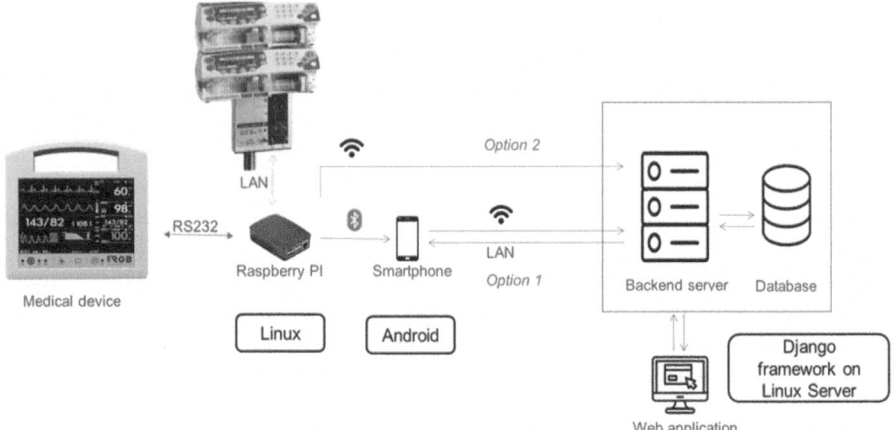

Fig. 2. Pilot 1 Architecture

Pilot 2 (Fig. 3), Cybersecurity for Telemedicine Platforms, will be conducted as an observational study, including patient participation. This pilot addresses critical vulnerabilities associated with connected medical devices (CMDs) and their gateways, focusing on ensuring the integrity of patient data transmitted to telemedicine platforms. As telemedicine's role expands in healthcare, protecting against data breaches, tampering, and misuse of medical devices becomes increasingly crucial. Notably, the pilot uniquely emphasises real-world applications and integration. Critical aspects of the pilot include:

- **Objective:** Ensuring the integrity of patient data transmitted to telemedicine platforms, safeguarding against data breaches and misuse of medical devices.
- **Significance:** With a growing reliance on telemedicine, this pilot addresses key cybersecurity concerns in healthcare, offering a comprehensive evaluation of the CYLCOMED toolbox.
- **Strategic Approach:** Simulated testing allows the assessment of sensitive components, ensuring the toolbox's reliability and effectiveness in both real and simulated scenarios.
- **Innovation and Adaptability:** By bringing developed tools into real-world applications, CYLCOMED demonstrates its commitment to innovation and adaptability in the evolving landscape of telemedicine cybersecurity.

The pilot involves enhancing the Mediaclinics Health Platform, focusing on paediatric patients. Clinicians will utilise the platform's remote monitoring capabilities to record and evaluate vital parameters from young patients. This approach strengthens cybersecurity and sets a precedent for secure and efficient telemedicine practices in healthcare.

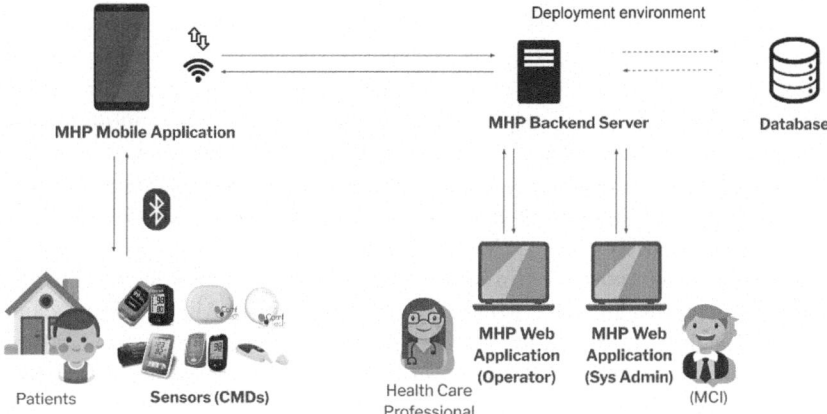

Fig. 3. MHP Architecture

5 Exploring Legal Implications and EU Regulations for Connected Medical Devices

Regulating cybersecurity, especially in the context of medical devices, is a complex challenge due to the specialised and fragmented nature of the legal framework (Chowdhury and Wessel 2012). The complexity of cybersecurity technology, such as the proposed CYLCOMED technology, arises from the intersection of various EU legislative frameworks and their potential applicability. Consequently, this complexity is compounded by the need to navigate both medical device regulations and cybersecurity laws (Biasin and Kamenjasevic 2020). When it comes to the legal requirements for the cybersecurity of medical devices, the EU laws establish a set of different requirements enshrined in the Medical Devices Regulation (MDR), In vitro Diagnostic Medical Devices (IVDR), the Cybersecurity Act (CSA), the Network and Information Systems Directive (NIS2), the General Data Protection Regulation (GDPR), the Radio Equipment Directive (RED) and recently adopted Artificial Intelligence Act (AI Act). The following subsections will provide a brief examination of these relevant legal frameworks.

5.1 Medical Device Regulation (MDR)

The MDR is the most crucial piece of legislation applicable to the cybersecurity of medical devices. The introduction of the MDR has emerged as a response to the risks and challenges posed by technological advancements in healthcare. In contrast to the previously repealed Medical Device Directive, the MDR imposes more rigorous requirements for bringing medical devices to the EU market or putting them into service inside of the EU. To ensure a high level of safety and performance of medical devices incorporating electronic programmable systems and software that is a medical device in itself, MDR requires a demonstration of compliance with the cybersecurity rules that are encompassed by the General and Safety Performance Requirements enlisted in Annex I (Article 5(2)).

According to Article 2(1) MDR, a medical device is defined as any instrument, apparatus, appliance, software, implant, reagent, material, or other article intended by the manufacturer to be used, alone or in combination, for human beings for one or more specific medical purposes. These purposes include diagnosis, prevention, monitoring, prediction, prognosis, treatment, alleviation of disease, investigation, replacement, or modification of anatomy or physiological/pathological processes or states. For instance, under the scope of the definition falls everything from plaster, disposable gloves to pacemakers and radiation systems (Malvehy et al. 2022).

To assist device manufacturers in adhering to the essential requirements in Annex I of the Medical Devices Regulation (MDR) concerning cybersecurity, the European Commission's Medical Device Coordination Group endorsed the Guidance on Cybersecurity for Medical Devices MDCG 2019-16 Rev.1 (MDCG Guidance). Being the first guidance on medical device cybersecurity, it marked a significant advancement in facilitating the implementation of MDR cybersecurity provisions. However, the medical device cybersecurity landscape is a dynamic field that has undergone significant changes since the MDCG Guidance endorsement in 2019. Scholars, including Biasin and Kamenjasevic (2020), have astutely identified areas for improvement in the MDCG Guidance. These include clarifying concepts such as joint responsibility and improving terminological coherence. These refinements are essential for the benefit of all stakeholders involved in medical device cybersecurity. The practical implementation of cybersecurity requirements outlined in the MDR has become more complex due to recent changes in the EU's regulatory frameworks that intersect with the medical device cybersecurity domain. Notably, introducing regulations like NIS2 has added an additional layer of intricacy to navigating and adhering to MDR cybersecurity provisions.

5.2 General Data Protection Regulation (GDPR)

The GDPR is particularly relevant to the cybersecurity of medical devices because these devices involve processing significant amounts of personal data, including sensitive data. The GDPR establishes rules for safeguarding individuals in processing their personal and sensitive data, specifically focusing on health-related data. As outlined in GDPR Article 25, one of the central requirements is the implementation of appropriate technical and organisational measures and necessary safeguards to ensure the practical application of data protection principles by design and default.

According to GDPR Article 25(1), data controllers and/or processors are mandated to establish appropriate technical and organisational measures proportional to the data processing risk. State-of-the-art criteria must be considered when implementing these measures. However, the term state-of-the-art is not precisely defined in the GDPR. In its Recital 78, the GDPR provides some examples of technical and organisational measures. However, the specific meaning of state-of-the-art remains open and subject to ongoing technological advancements, as the European Data Protection Board (EDPB) acknowledges in its Guidelines on Article 25 Data Protection by Design and by Default. While the GDPR obliges the data controllers and/or processors to ground the implementation of these measures on the risk-based approach, considering the current technological progress, the practical implementation leaves room for different interpretations of what constitutes the state-of-the-art.

5.3 Network and Information Systems Directive (NISD)

The Network and Information Security Directive (NISD) 2016/1148/EU is considered to be the first piece of EU-wide cybersecurity legislation, which aimed, among other things, to build cybersecurity capabilities across the Union and mitigate threats to network and information systems (Markopoulou et al. 2019). Despite its significant achievements, such as a positive shift in the cybersecurity framework and improved cyber resilience of public and private entities, the European Commission's Impact assessment (2020) on the NIS Directive has demonstrated its limitations over time. Due to identified shortcomings in implementing the NIS Directive, it was repealed by the NIS2 Directive, which introduced various novelties and expanded the scope of its application. While the repealed Directive has encompassed the healthcare sector, the NIS2 expands its scope of application to new entities. It applies to manufacturers of medical devices, imposing additional cybersecurity requirements established in the NIS2 Directive on these entities.

NIS2 differentiates two categories of entities that fall within the scope of the Directive: essential entities and important entities listed in Annexes I and II of the NIS 2 Directive. The distinction between them is based on the criticality of essential entities and important entities concerning their sector or the type of service they provide, their size, and a compliance obligation. These will be subject to cybersecurity risk management and reporting obligations, and they will be supervised, to different degrees, by the competent authorities. With reporting obligation, it has been acknowledged that certain malicious attacks can invoke the simultaneous application of MDR's and NIS2's provisions, thus causing legal uncertainty and overlap (Biasin and Kamenjasevic 2020). However, the specific requirements mandated by the NIS2 are still ambiguous, as the detailed requirements of the NIS2 Directive are to be released by October 2024. More specifically, Member States shall adopt and publish the measures necessary to comply with this Directive by 17 October 2024 (Article 41).

5.4 Cyber Security Act (CSA)

The Cyber Security Act (CSA) aims to ensure the proper functioning of the EU's internal market by reaching a high level of cybersecurity of network and information systems, communication networks, services, and devices within the Union. CSA establishes the first EU-wide cybersecurity certification framework to ensure a common cybersecurity certification approach in the European internal market and ultimately improve cybersecurity in a broad range of digital products and services. Certification is seen as vital for increasing the trust and security of ICT products, ICT services or ICT processes (CSA Recital 69). Besides, cybersecurity certification aims to overcome the fragmentation and overlapping of national cybersecurity certification schemes. Furthermore, it strives to enable a harmonised approach at the Union level to European cybersecurity certification schemes to create a single digital market for ICT products, ICT services, and ICT processes. However, it is essential to note that according to the CSA Article 56(2), cybersecurity certification is voluntary unless otherwise specified by EU or Member State regulations. If some member states were to require a mandatory cybersecurity certification, it would mean that manufacturers would have to obtain a cybersecurity certificate for a device to be marketed within a particular Member State. However, this requirement may not be necessary in other Member States, causing inconsistency across countries (Biasin and Kamenjasevic 2020). In such cases, manufacturers of devices that obtained CE marking might be obliged to undergo an additional certification process, thus causing duplication of requirements and additional costs. Additionally, the recently adopted AI Act introduces a certification mechanism, which will add an additional layer of complexity to this domain.

5.5 Radio Equipment Directive (RED)

The Radio Equipment Directive (RED) establishes a regulatory framework for making available on the EU market and putting radio equipment into service. Certain types of medical devices (such as pacemakers or implantable cardioverter defibrillators) are likely to fall under the scope of the Directive and thus be subject to its security requirements. All internet-connected radio equipment that is Wi-Fi, Bluetooth, LTE, 5G, or GPS enabled falls under the scope of RED. Consequently, the RED applies to medical devices if they include components such as Wi-Fi or Bluetooth modules, which means that, apart from meeting stringent MDR requirements, medical device manufacturers will need to comply with RED, conduct conformity assessment under its rules, and declare conformity with RED, in addition to the MDR. Additionally, the Commission adopted a Delegated Act of the Radio Equipment Directive, which aims to increase the level of cybersecurity, personal data protection and privacy for specific categories of radio equipment. The Delegated Regulation has brought clarity and relief to medical device manufacturers as it excludes medical devices from its scope regarding cybersecurity requirements (Article 2(1a)).

5.6 AI Act

The AI Act, a landmark piece of legislation regulating artificial intelligence technologies, was published in the European Journal on July 12, 2024. Its primary goal is to mitigate risks to health, safety, and fundamental rights associated with AI technologies. This comprehensive legislation, with its broad scope of application, including the medical device sector, is set to significantly impact the industry.

However, it is worth noting that AI is not a novelty in healthcare settings. Artificial intelligence has made significant inroads into the medical field, enhancing diagnostic accuracy, personalising treatment plans, and improving patient outcomes. In the medical devices domain, AI-driven technologies have been deployed for advanced imaging, predictive analytics, and even robotic surgeries. AI medical devices are subject to stringent requirements laid down by MDR. Moreover, many AI medical devices have been CE-marked under the now-repealed Medical Device Directive (Choi et al. 2022). However, some scholars have raised serious concerns that due to the unique nature of AI, MDR falls short of regulating these unique characteristics (Li et al. 2023; Mkwashi and Brass 2022).

Upon enforcing the AI Act, medical device manufacturers will be required to comply with additional obligations stipulated by the AI Act, in conjunction with the existing MDR requirements, which will undoubtedly add another layer of complexity to the already complex regulatory landscape. Namely, most AI medical device software will fall under the scope of high-risk AI systems (Article 6(1)) since all medical device software class IIa and higher needs to undergo a third-party conformity assessment. Some of the new requirements refer to data and data governance (Article 10), Record-keeping (Article 12) and Human oversight (Article 14), to mention just a few. Consequently, medical device manufacturers, apart from MDR requirements, will have to comply with requirements for high-risk AI systems established by the AI Act, which will undoubtedly significantly affect the MedTech industry, raising overall compliance costs. Many scholars have already highlighted potential duplication and inconsistency in the interplay between the MDR and the AI Act (Choi et al. 2022; Biasin et al. 2023b). Moreover, all applicable requirements are outlined at a high level, lacking detailed specifications for their implementation. To avoid legal uncertainty, it is crucial to clarify the relationship between the MDR and the AI Act and the practical implementation of high-level requirements. In this regard, industrial standards and MDCG guidance are expected to play crucial roles in facilitating compliance. Although the European Commission has issued a standardisation request to the European Committee for Standardisation (CEN) and the European Committee for Electrotechnical Standardisation (CENELEC) to support safe and trustworthy artificial intelligence, the timeline for developing these standards remains uncertain due to the lengthy and complex nature of the process.

While the AI Act addresses cybersecurity through several recitals and articles, it is not cybersecurity legislation per se. Its Recital 76 AI Act acknowledges that cybersecurity is fundamental in safeguarding AI systems against attempts by malicious entities to alter their utilisation, behaviour, and performance or to compromise their security attributes by exploiting system vulnerabilities. AI cybersecurity is encompassed within Article 15 of the AI Act, although not as an individual requirement, but integrated with considerations of accuracy and robustness. AI Act Article 15(1) prescribes that high-risk AI systems shall be designed and developed in such a way that they achieve an appropriate level of accuracy, robustness, and cybersecurity and that they perform consistently in those respects throughout their lifecycle. However, their practical implementation is still ambiguous since the cybersecurity requirements are outlined in broad terms. Additionally, despite provisions addressing cybersecurity, some scholars (Biasin et al. 2023b) have noted that the AI Act does not explicitly reference the Cybersecurity Act's definition of cybersecurity. This omission is significant, as it would establish a stronger connection to individual cybersecurity protection.

6 Conclusion

The health sector faces persistent threats, with patient data, including electronic health records, ranking as the primary target. Despite increased attention and policy efforts, the healthcare industry lags in terms of cybersecurity maturity and competence compared to sectors like industrial and financial.

This article emphasises the critical importance of cybersecurity in healthcare, particularly for CMDs and the IoMT. With healthcare's increasing digitisation, CMDs are exposed to various cyber threats that can compromise patient safety, data privacy, and operational integrity.

Additionally, this article delves into the background of the proposed CYLCOMED cybersecurity solution situated within an interdisciplinary research paradigm. It further aims to analyse the leading cybersecurity challenges in the healthcare sector and introduce the ambitious goal of CYLCOMED cybersecurity solutions, which aims to strengthen the cybersecurity of connected medical devices. Following CYLCOMED as an example, the article explores the regulatory landscape, examining how EU legal frameworks set standards for cybersecurity in medical devices. The legal landscape surrounding cybersecurity in the EU is complex, involving various frameworks such as the Medical Device Regulation (MDR), General Data Protection Regulation (GDPR), Network and Information Systems Directive (NISD), Cyber Security Act (CSA), Radio Equipment Directive (RED) and recently adopted AI Act.

Navigating these legal frameworks presents challenges, with recent changes such as NIS2 and AI Act adding complexity to the practical implementation of MDR cybersecurity requirements. The GDPR is particularly relevant due to the vast amount of personal data processed by medical devices, emphasising the need for appropriate technical and organisational measures.

Although the CYLCOMED project's architecture aligns with these regulations, the evolving legal landscape and the dynamic nature of medical devices and cybersecurity necessitate ongoing adaptation. Challenges persist, such as clarifying joint responsibility and improving terminological coherence, to mention just a few.

In conclusion, CYLCOMED's proactive approach, incorporating a robust cybersecurity toolbox and real-world pilot implementations, aligns with the imperative to address the evolving challenges in connected medical device cybersecurity. Ongoing legal developments add layers of complexity, emphasising the need for continuous adaptation and collaboration across stakeholders in the healthcare and cybersecurity domains.

Acknowledgement. CYLCOMED [Cyber securitY tooLbox for COnnected MEdical Devices] project has received funding from the European Union's (Horizon Europe) research and innovation programme under grant agreement No 101095542.

Data Availability. No data was used for the research described in this article.

Declaration of Competing Interest. Dusko Milojevic and Maja Nisevic declare not to have any conflict of interest.

References

Al-Qahtani, A.F., Cresci, S.: The COVID-19 scamdemic: a survey of phishing attacks and their countermeasures during COVID-19. IET Inf. Secur. **16**(5), 324–345 (2022). https://doi.org/10.1049/ise2.12073

Anderson, S., Fagerberg, J.: "mHealth and Home Monitoring". Berg Insight (2023). https://www.berginsight.com/mhealth-and-home-monitoring

Biasin, E., Kamenjasevic, E., Rosager Ludvigsen, K.: Cybersecurity of AI medical devices: risks, legislation, and challenges. arXiv e-prints, arXiv-2303 (2023a)

Biasin, E., Yasar, B., Kamenjasevic, E.: New cybersecurity requirements for medical devices in the EU: the forthcoming European health data space, data act, and artificial intelligence act. Law Tech. Hum. **5**, 43 (2023b). https://doi.org/10.5204/lthj.3068

Biasin, E., Kamenjasevic, E.: Cybersecurity of medical devices: regulatory challenges in the EU (2020). https://doi.org/10.2139/ssrn.3855491

Chowdhury, N., Wessel, R.A.: Conceptualising multilevel regulation in the EU: a legal translation of multilevel governance? Eur. Law J. **18**(3), 335–357 (2012). https://doi.org/10.1111/j.1468-0386.2012.00603.x

CISO Global. Most Dangerous Hacked Medical Devices (2018). https://www.alpinesecurity.com/blog/most-dangerous-hacked-medical-devices/

Choi, W., Van Eck, M., Cécile van der, H.H.T., Vollebregt, E.: Legal analysis: European legislative proposal draft AI act and MDR/IVDR. Hooghiemstra and Partners (2022). Report+analysis+AI+act+-+MDR+and+IVDR.pdf

Commission Delegated Regulation (EU) 2022/30 of 29 October 2021 supplementing Directive 2014/53/EU of the European Parliament and of the Council with regard to the application of the essential requirements referred to in Article 3(3), points (d), (e) and (f), of that Directive (Text with EEA relevance). EUR-Lex - 32022R0030 - EN - EUR-Lex (europa.eu) (2021)

Cyber Security Policy. "Securing Cyber Resilience in Health and Care: Progress Update 2018". London: Department of Health & Social Care; Securing cyber resilience in health and care: September 2018 update (publishing.service.gov.uk) (2018)

Evans, M., He, Y., Maglaras, L., Janicke, H.: HEART-IS: a novel technique for evaluating human error-related information security incidents. Comput. Secur. **80**, 74–89 (2018). https://doi.org/10.1016/j.cose.2018.09.002

European Commission. "Impact assessment Proposal for directive on measures for high common level of cybersecurity across the Union". Impact assessment Proposal for directive on measures for high common level of cybersecurity across the Union | Shaping Europe's digital future (europa.eu) (2020)

European Data Protection Board (EDPB). "Guidelines 4/2019 on Article 25 Data Protection by Design and Default". Guidelines 4/2019 on Article 25 Data Protection by Design and by Default | European Data Protection Board (europa.eu) (2019)

European Data Protection Board (EDBP). Administrative fine imposed on psychotherapy centre Vastaamo for data protection violations. Administrative fine imposed on psychotherapy centre Vastaamo for data protection violations | European Data Protection Board (europa. eu) (2022)

European Parliament. 2021. The EU's Cybersecurity Strategy for the Digital Decade. Texts dopted - The EU's Cybersecurity Strategy for the Digital Decade - Thursday, 10 June 2021 (europa.eu)

European Union Agency for Cybersecurity (ENISA). "NIS Investments 2022" (2022). https://www.enisa.europa.eu/publications/nis-investments-2022

European Union Agency for Cybersecurity (ENISA). "Threat Landscape for Ransomware Attacks 2022" (2022). https://www.enisa.europa.eu/publications/enisa-threat-landscape-for-ransomware-attacks

The European Union Agency for Cybersecurity (ENISA). "Health Threat Landscape" (2023a). https://www.enisa.europa.eu/publications/health-threat-landscape

European Union Agency for Cybersecurity (ENISA). "ENISA Threat Landscape 2023" (2023b). https://www.enisa.europa.eu/publications/enisa-threat-landscape-2023

European Union Agency for Cybersecurity (ENISA). "Foresight 2030 Threats" (2023c). https://www.enisa.europa.eu/publications/foresight-2030-threats

European Union Agency for Cybersecurity (ENISA). "Cybersecurity Skills Development in the EU" (2020). https://www.enisa.europa.eu/publications/the-status-of-cyber-security-education-in-the-european-union

European Union. Regulation (EU) 2024/1689 of the European Parliament and of the Council of 13 June 2024 laying down harmonised rules on artificial intelligence and amending Regulations (EC) No 300/2008, (EU) No 167/2013, (EU) No 168/2013, (EU) 2018/858, (EU) 2018/1139 and (EU) 2019/2144 and Directives 2014/90/EU, (EU) 2016/797 and (EU) 2020/1828 (Artificial Intelligence Act) (2024)

European Union. Regulation (EU) 2023/2854 of the European Parliament and of the Council of 13 December 2023 on harmonised rules on fair access to and use of data and amending Regulation (EU) 2017/2394 and Directive (EU) 2020/1828 (Data Act) (2023)

European Union. Regulation (EU) 2019/881 of the European Parliament and of the Council of 17 April 2019 on ENISA (the European Union Agency for Cybersecurity) and on information and communications technology cybersecurity certification and repealing Regulation (EU) No 526/2013 (Cybersecurity Act). EUR-Lex - 32019R0881 - EN - EUR-Lex (europa.eu) (2019)

European Union. Regulation (EU) 2017/745 of the European Parliament and of the Council of 5 April 2017 on medical devices, amending Directive 2001/83/EC, Regulation (EC) No 178/2002 and Regulation (EC) No 1223/2009 and repealing Council Directives 90/385/EEC and 93/42/EEC (Text with EEA relevance.). Available at EUR-Lex - 32017R0745 - EN - EUR-Lex (europa.eu) (2017)

European Union. Directive (EU) 2022/2555 of the European Parliament and of the Council of 14 December 2022 on measures for a high common level of cybersecurity across the Union, amending Regulation (EU) No 910/2014 and Directive (EU) 2018/1972, and repealing Directive (EU) 2016/1148 (NIS 2 Directive) (Text with EEA relevance). Available at EUR-Lex - 32022L2555 - EN - EUR-Lex (europa.eu) (2022)

European Union. Directive (EU) 2016/1148 of the European Parliament and of the Council of 6 July 2016 concerning measures for a high common level of security of network and information systems across the Union OJ L 194 (NISD). Available at EUR-Lex - 32016L1148 - EN - EUR-Lex (europa.eu) (2016)

European Union. Directive 2014/53/EU of the European Parliament and of the Council of 16 April 2014 on the harmonisation of the laws of the Member States relating to the making available on the market of radio equipment and repealing Directive 1999/5/EC Text with EEA relevance. EUR-Lex - 32014L0053 - EN - EUR-Lex (europa.eu) (2014)

European Data Protection Supervisor (EDPS). "Opinion 23/2022 on the Proposal for a Regulation of the European Parliament and of the Council on horizontal cybersecurity requirements for products with digital elements and amending Regulation (EU) 2019/1020" (2022). https://edps.europa.eu/system/files/2022-11/2022-0921_d2649_opinion_en.pdf

Federal Bureau of Investigation (FBI). "Internet Crime Report 2023". 2023_IC3Report.pdf (2023)

O'Neill Patrick, H.: Ransomware did not kill a German Hospital patient. MIT Technology Review (2020). Accesse 12 Nov 2020. https://www.technologyreview.com/2020/11/12/1012015/ransomware-did-not-kill-a-german-hospital-patient/

Huang, C., Wang, J., Wang, S., Zhang, Y.: Internet of medical things: a systematic review. Neurocomputing **557**, 126719 (2023). https://doi.org/10.1016/j.neucom.2023.126719

Humer, C., Finkle, J.: Your medical record is worth more to hackers than your credit card. Accessed 24 Sept 2014. https://www.reuters.com/article/us-cybersecurity-hospitals-idUSKCN0HJ21I20140924/

IBM Security. "Cost of a Data Breach Report 2023" (2023). https://www.ibm.com/reports/data-breach

International Medical Device Regulators Forum (IMDRF). "Principles and Practices for the Cybersecurity of Legacy Medical Devices". IMDRF Principles and Practices of Cybersecurity for Legacy Medical Devices Final (N70).pdf (2023)

ISC2. "CYBERSECURITY WORKFORCE STUDY". Cybersecurity Workforce Study (isc2.org) (2023)

Javaid, M., Haleem, A., Singh, R.P., Suman, R.: Towards insighting cybersecurity for healthcare domains: a comprehensive review of recent practices and trends. Cyber Secur. Appl. **1**, 100016 (2023). https://doi.org/10.1016/j.csa.2023.100016

Kotz, D., Gunter, C.A., Kumar, S., Weiner, J.P.: Privacy and security in mobile health: a research agenda. Computer **49**(6), 22–30 (2016). https://doi.org/10.1109/MC.2016.185

Li, P., Williams, R., Gilbert, S., Anderson, S.: Regulating artificial intelligence and machine learning-enabled medical devices in Europe and the United Kingdom. Law Tech. Hum. **5**, 94 (2023). https://doi.org/10.5204/lthj.3073

Levy-Loboda, T., Sheetrit, E., Liberty, I.F., Haim, A., Nissim, N.: Personalized insulin dose manipulation attack and its detection using interval-based temporal patterns and machine learning algorithms. J. Biomed. Inf. **132**, 104129 (2022). https://doi.org/10.1016/j.jbi.2022.104129

Mkwashi, A., Brass, I.: The Future of Medical Device Regulation and Standards: Dealing with Critical Challenges for Connected, Intelligent Medical Devices. PETRAS National Centre of Excellent in IoT Systems Cybersecurity, London (2022a). https://doi.org/10.5281/zenodo.7054048

Malvehy, J., Ginsberg, R., Sampietro-Colom, L., Ficapal, J., Combalia, M., Svedenhag, P.: New regulation of medical devices in the EU: impact in dermatology. J. Eur. Acad. Dermatol. Venereol. **36**(3), 360–364 (2022). https://doi.org/10.1111/jdv.17830

Markopoulou, D., Papakonstantinou, V., De Hert, P.: The new EU cybersecurity framework: the NIS directive, ENISA's role and the general data protection regulation. Comput. Law Secur. Rev. **35**(6), 105336 (2019). https://doi.org/10.1016/j.clsr.2019.06.007

Medical Device Coordination Group. December, 2019. "Guidance on Cybersecurity for medical devices". (MDCG 2019–16 Rev.1). Available at: md_cybersecurity_en.pdf (europa.eu)

Medtronic. "Security Bulletin". Accessed 27 June 2019. https://global.medtronic.com/xg-en/product-security/security-bulletins/minimed-508-paradigm.html

Mkwashi, A., Brass, I.: The future of medical device regulation and standards: dealing with critical challenges for connected, intelligent medical devices. PETRAS National Centre of Excellent in IoT Systems Cybersecurity, London (2022B). https://doi.org/10.2139/ssrn.4226057

National Audit Office. "Report-Value for money; Investigation: WannaCry Cyber Attack and the NHS". Investigation: WannaCry cyber attack and the NHS - NAO report (2017)

National Institute of Standards and Technology (NIST). "Supporting the Growth and Sustainment of the Nation's Cybersecurity Workforce: Building the Foundation for a More Secure American Future". Supporting the Growth and Sustainment of the Nation's Cybersecurity Workforce | CISA (2020)

Pattnaik, N., et al.: It's more than just money: the real-world harms from ransomware attacks. In: Furnell, S., Clarke, N. (eds.) Human Aspects of Information Security and Assurance: 17th IFIP WG 11.12 International Symposium, HAISA 2023, Kent, UK, July 4–6, 2023, Proceedings, pp. 261–274. Springer Nature Switzerland, Cham (2023). https://doi.org/10.1007/978-3-031-38530-8_21

Papageorgiou, A., Strigkos, M., Politou, E., Alepis, E., Solanas, A., Patsakis, C.: Security and privacy analysis of mobile health applications: the alarming state of practice. IEEE Access **6**, 9390–9403 (2018). https://doi.org/10.1109/ACCESS.2018.2799522

Perakslis, E.D.: Cybersecurity in health care. N. Engl. J. Med. **371**(5), 395–397 (2014)

Piggin, R.: Cybersecurity of medical devices: addressing patient safety and the security of patient health information. BSI Group, Macquarie Park, Australia, White Paper (2017)

Pollack, Rick. "Impact and Aftermath of the Change Healthcare Cyberattack: Insights from the AHA". Health Management. April 4, 2024. impact-and-aftermath-of-the-change-healthcare-cyberattack-insights-from-the-aha.pdf

Porter, S.: Cyberattack on Czech hospital forces tech shutdown during coronavirus outbreak. HealthCare IT News. Cyberattack on Czech hospital forces tech shutdown during coronavirus outbreak | Healthcare IT News (2020)

Proposal for a REGULATION OF THE EUROPEAN PARLIAMENT AND OF THE COUNCIL on horizontal cybersecurity requirements for products with digital elements and amending Regulation (EU) 2019/1020. EUR-Lex - 52022PC0454 - EN - EUR-Lex (europa.eu)

Proposal for a REGULATION OF THE EUROPEAN PARLIAMENT AND OF THE COUNCIL LAYING DOWN HARMONISED RULES ON ARTIFICIAL INTELLIGENCE (ARTIFICIAL INTELLIGENCE ACT) AND AMENDING CERTAIN UNION LEGISLATIVE ACTS. EUR-Lex - 52021PC0206 - EN - EUR-Lex (europa.eu)

Quinn, P.: The EU commission's risky choice for a non-risk based strategy on assessment of medical devices. Comput. Law Secur. Rev. **33**(3), 361–370 (2017). https://doi.org/10.1016/j.clsr.2017.03.019

Raina MacIntyre, C., et al.: Converging and emerging threats to health security. Environ. Syst. Decis. **38**, 198–207 (2018). https://doi.org/10.1007/s10669-017-9667-0

Rak, R.: Internet of healthcare: opportunities and legal challenges in Internet of things-enabled telehealth ecosystems. In: Proceedings of the 14th International Conference on Theory and Practice of Electronic Governance, pp. 481–484 (2021). https://doi.org/10.1145/3494193.3494260

Ray, A.: Introduction to medical device cybersecurity. Cybersecur. Connect. Med. Dev., 1–28 (2021). https://doi.org/10.1016/B978-0-12-818262-8.00004-8

Schwab, K.: The fourth industrial revolution. Crown Currency (2017)

Shenoy, A., Appel, J.M.: Safeguarding confidentiality in electronic health records. Camb. Q. Healthc. Ethics **26**(2), 337–341 (2017). https://doi.org/10.1017/S0963180116000931

Silver, J.K., Binder, D.S., Zubcevik, N., Zafonte, R.D.: Healthcare hackathons provide educational and innovation opportunities: a case study and best practice recommendations. J. Med. Syst. **40**, 1–7 (2016). https://doi.org/10.1007/s10916-016-0532-3

Slabodkin, G.: Legacy medical devices, growing hacker threats create perfect storm of cybersecurity risks. MEDTECHDIVE (2021). https://www.medtechdive.com/news/legacy-medical-devices-growing-hacker-threats-create-medtech-cyber-risks/602157/

Srivastava, N., Pandey, P.: Internet of things (IoT): applications, trends, issues and challenges. Mater. Today: Proc. **69**, 587–591 (2022). https://doi.org/10.1016/j.matpr.2022.09.490

Stack, B.: Here's how much your personal information is selling for on the dark web (2017). Here's How Much Your Personal Information Is Selling for on the Dark Web - Experian

Takahashi, D.: Insulin pump hacker says vendor Medtronic is ignoring security risk. VentureBeat (2011). https://venturebeat.com/business/insulin-pump-hacker-says-vendor-medtronic-is-ignoring-security-risk/

The Healthcare Information and Management Systems Society (HIMSS). Healthcare Cybersecurity Survey (2022). https://www.himss.org/sites/hde/files/media/file/2023/04/17/2022-himss-cybersecurity-survey-x.pdf

The White House. "Executive Order on Improving the Nation's Cybersecurity" (2021). https://www.whitehouse.gov/briefing-room/presidential-actions/2021/05/12/executive-order-on-improving-the-nations-cybersecurity/

The White House. National Cybersecurity Strategy (2023). https://www.whitehouse.gov/wp-content/uploads/2023/03/National-Cybersecurity-Strategy-2023.pdf

Ursula von der Leyen. Speech "State of the Union 2021". September 15 2021, Strasbourg. State of the Union Address by President von der Leyen (europa.eu) (2021)

Waegemann, C.P.: IT security: developing a response to increasing risks. Int. J. Biomed. Comput. **43**(1–2), 5–8 (1996). https://doi.org/10.1016/s0020-7101(96)01220-2

Walker-Roberts, S., Hammoudeh, M., Dehghantanha, A.: A systematic review of the availability and efficacy of countermeasures to internal threats in healthcare critical infrastructure. IEEE Access **6**, 25167–25177 (2018). https://doi.org/10.1109/ACCESS.2021.3109886

Weber, R.H., Studer, E.: Cybersecurity in the internet of things: legal aspects. Comput. Law Secur. Rev. **32**(5), 715–728 (2016). https://doi.org/10.1016/j.clsr.2016.07.002

Williams, P.A., Woodward, A.J.: Cybersecurity vulnerabilities in medical devices: a complex environment and multifaceted problem. Med. Dev. Evid. Res., 305–316 (2015). https://doi.org/10.2147/MDER.S50048

Wirth, A.: Hardly ever a dull moment: the ongoing cyberthreats of 2017. Biomed. Instrum. Technol. **51**(5), 431–433 (2017). https://doi.org/10.2345/0899-8205-51.5.431

World Economic Forum (WEF). The Global Risks Report 2024 (2024). Global Risks Report 2024 | World Economic Forum | World Economic Forum

Yaqoob, T., Abbas, H., Atiquzzaman, M.: Security vulnerabilities, attacks, countermeasures, and regulations of networked medical devices—a review. IEEE Commun. Surv. Tutor. **21**(4), 3723–3768 (2019). https://doi.org/10.1109/COMST.2019.2914094

Yigzaw, K.Y., et al.: Health data security and privacy: challenges and solutions for the future. In: Roadmap to Successful Digital Health Ecosystems, pp. 335–362 (2022). https://doi.org/10.1016/B978-0-12-823413-6.00014-8

A Study and Assessment of the Importance of Cybersecurity in the Internet of Things for Healthcare Wearables

Mohammed Ridha Faisa Faisal[✉]

Computer Engineering, Ibn Khaldun University College, Baghdad, Iraq
drengmrf@gmail.com

Abstract. The rapid progress in the field of e-health services has become more and more highlighting the importance of information security in the healthcare sector. Healthcare organizations are facing increasing cyber threats, as innovative medical devices and healthcare applications used to treat patients have become attractive targets for cyber attacks. When hacking networks, attackers can disable vital services or encrypt data using ransomware, which leads to interruptions of operations and large payments for their restoration, especially since healthcare services are highly time-dependent. In addition, these attacks may result in serious security risks, such as hacking network-connected devices, causing errors with the distribution of medicines, or changing the functions of medical devices in an unsafe way.

Academic research reveals the prevalence of cyber threats in the healthcare sector and how existing vulnerabilities can be exploited. The increase in data collection processes and access points in healthcare systems makes patient data a valuable target for cybercriminals. The collection of patients' health data from various sources, such as hospital and laboratory records, insurance information, fitness applications, tracking devices, and health portals, complicates data security and increases security vulnerabilities.

In this context, implementing an effective cybersecurity strategy in the healthcare sector is a critical requirement to protect the integrity of data and prevent potential breaches. The use of cybersecurity technologies ensures the protection of health data, thus ensuring both patient privacy and the uninterrupted provision of healthcare services. As a result, strengthening cybersecurity in the healthcare sector necessitates the development of defense mechanisms against increasing threats for both institutions and individuals.

Keywords: Cybersecurity · IoT · Healthcare Wearables

1 Introduction

The healthcare sector is facing a significant challenge in terms of cybersecurity at a time when dependence on technology is increasing. While computer-aided healthcare systems and internet-based devices greatly facilitate the functioning of healthcare institutions, they also bring with them data security risks. Innovative technologies such as electronic health records (EHR), medical devices, patient monitoring systems and mobile health applications used in healthcare delivery have become the target of cybercriminals because they contain sensitive data [17].

In today's world, patient information is considered one of the most valuable types of data. Hackers can steal this data and commit crimes such as ransomware, identity theft and fraud. The healthcare sector has a broader security responsibility compared to many other industries, as data breaches in this sector can cause not only financial losses but also harm human life. Therefore, ensuring cybersecurity in healthcare is of critical importance in terms of protecting patient safety and data integrity [18].

2 Wearable Health Devices and the Spread of IoT Technology

With the digitalization of healthcare, wearable health devices (wearables) have become rapidly widespread. Devices such as smart watches, fitness trackers, heart rhythm monitoring systems, and blood pressure monitors allow individuals to continuously monitor their health status. These devices collect individual health information and provide real-time data to users and healthcare professionals. However, since these devices mostly transmit data over the internet, they are highly vulnerable to cybersecurity threats [19].

The integration of wearable devices into the Internet of Things (IoT) ecosystem has increased the quality of healthcare services while increasing security threats to the same extent. Since the data collected through these devices is shared with healthcare systems, cloud storage solutions, and even third-party applications, this information must be stored and processed securely. Cybersecurity deficiencies in wearable devices not only endanger patient privacy, but can also lead to incorrect treatment decisions [20].

Benefits and Applications of Wearable Devices
Wearable devices offer substantial benefits, allowing individuals to manage their health without frequent hospital visits [1]. They also enable healthcare providers to access continuous data on patients, improving diagnostic accuracy and helping in treatment decisions (Table 1).

Table 1. Types of Wearable Health Devices, Their Applications, and Benefits:

Device Type	Application Areas	Benefits
Smartwatches	Heart rate, steps, sleep	Daily health tracking, fitness activity logging
Fitness Trackers	Activity, calorie counting	Physical activity monitoring, lifestyle support
Heart Rhythm Monitors	Heart rate tracking	Continuous monitoring for heart patients
Blood Pressure Monitors	Blood pressure measurement	Convenient tracking for hypertension patients

2.1 The Role and Importance of Wearable Devices in the IoT Ecosystem

Wearable health devices, integrated into the IoT ecosystem, have improved the quality of healthcare services. Operating within this ecosystem, wearable devices not only enable users to track their health but also share data with healthcare systems, cloud storage solutions, and even third-party applications [21].

Contributions of IoT Integration to Healthcare Services

IoT-enabled wearable devices allow healthcare professionals to monitor patients remotely and provide timely interventions in emergency situations. For example, a heart rhythm monitor can alert medical personnel if it detects a critical irregularity in the user's heart rate (Fig. 1).

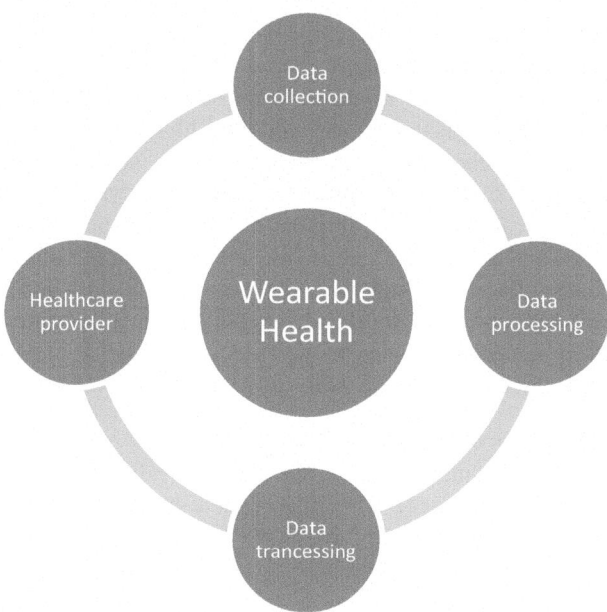

Fig. 1. The Role of IoT-Based Wearable Health Devices in the IoT Ecosystem and Data Flow [16].

1. **Data Collection:** Devices like smartwatches and blood pressure monitors collect health data.
2. **Data Processing:** Data is analyzed through the device itself or connected applications.
3. **Data Transmission:** Information is transmitted to cloud storage or healthcare providers.
4. **Healthcare Provider Access:** Medical personnel can access patient data remotely.

2.2 Cybersecurity Threats to Wearable Devices

The fact that most wearable devices transmit data over the internet makes them vulnerable to cybersecurity threats. Security vulnerabilities in wearable devices can expose sensitive health information and may even lead to incorrect medical decisions. Common security issues in wearable devices include weak encryption, insufficient physical security, and inadequate software updates [2] (Table 2).

Table 2. Common Cybersecurity Threats to Wearable Devices and Their Impact

Cybersecurity Threat	Description	Impact
Lack of Data Encryption	Health data is transmitted without encryption	Exposure of personal data
Insufficient Updates	Devices lack regular security updates	Persistent vulnerabilities
Weak Physical Security	Devices are prone to loss or theft	Unauthorized access to personal data

Real-Life Examples of Cybersecurity Threats
For instance, if health data is transmitted over an insecure network, it can be intercepted by unauthorized parties, potentially risking patient privacy. This can also lead to data manipulation, which may affect treatment decisions based on inaccurate information.

2.3 Necessary Security Measures for Wearable Devices

To ensure the security of wearable devices, several measures can be implemented. High-level encryption, multi-factor authentication, and regular security updates are essential. Additionally, users should be educated on proper security practices for device usage (Table 3).

Table 3. Recommended Security Measures for Wearable Devices and Their Benefits

Security Measure	Description	Benefits
Strong Encryption	Using AES, RSA encryption methods	Prevents unauthorized access to data
Multi-Factor Authentication	Verifies user identity	Reduces risk of unauthorized access
Regular Security Updates	Software and firmware updates	Protects against newly identified vulnerabilities

User Awareness and Training
It's also essential to educate users on secure practices, such as connecting to trusted networks instead of public Wi-Fi and understanding what to do if a device is lost or stolen [3].

2.4 Secure Data Sharing Within the IoT Ecosystem

Data sharing is a key component within the IoT ecosystem. The health data gathered by wearable devices is frequently shared with healthcare providers, cloud storage systems, and third-party applications. Therefore, it's crucial that data is encrypted and accessible only to authorized users.

Protocols for Secure Data Sharing

Secure communication protocols such as SSL/TLS are essential to protect health data as it travels through various points in the system. They ensure the security of this data and prevent any attempt to intercept or access it in an unauthorized way [5] (Table 4).

Table 4. Recommended Security Protocols for IoT-Based Wearable Devices

Protocol	Description	Application
SSL/TLS	Secure data transfer protocol	Health data transmission
HTTPS	Secure web-based data sharing	Health application communication
Advanced Encryption Standard	Strong encryption standard	Data transmission from device to cloud

Wearable health devices provide users with the ability to monitor their health condition well and appropriately, as well as help doctors and healthcare personnel with more accurate data for diagnosis and treatment. However, the integration of these devices within the IoT ecosystem introduces potential security risks. In order to realize the full benefits of wearable devices, high and strong security measures should be imposed, as well as users should be informed about how to use them safely. The rapid growth in this segment largely depends on the commitment to cybersecurity by both device manufacturers and users [7].

3 Security Risks of IoT-Based Health Devices

Existing IoT-based health devices offer significant advantages to the healthcare sector, as they can contain security vulnerabilities that in turn pose a risk to these devices. The fact that wearable devices that connect to the internet allow intruders and cybercriminals to indirectly access these devices and thus steal personal health information. For example, heart monitors or insulin pumps can be manipulated by cybercriminals, thereby endangering the patient's life.

The security vulnerabilities of these devices are not limited to theft of personal data. They can also result in changes to the functions of healthcare devices, incorrect data transmission, or rendering the devices dysfunctional. In this context, strengthening the security protocols of IoT devices is of great importance in preventing cyberattacks in the healthcare sector [10].

3.1 Unauthorized Access and Data Theft

Wearable IoT health devices are designed to collect and transmit highly sensitive personal health information over the internet, which cybercriminals can target. Hackers might exploit vulnerabilities in device software, unsecured network connections, or even data storage systems. Unauthorized access allows attackers to obtain personal data like heart rates, glucose levels, physical activity metrics, and other intimate health information. This data is valuable not only for the person it belongs to but also for potential misuse in identity theft, blackmail, or insurance fraud [8].

3.2 Manipulation of Critical Medical Devices

Wearable devices that play a critical role in patient care, like heart monitors and insulin pumps, are especially concerning when it comes to cybersecurity. If attackers gain access to these devices, they can potentially alter the device's functions, leading to inaccurate or manipulated data. This could cause serious health complications, for instance:

- **Heart Monitors**: Malicious tampering could disrupt a device's ability to accurately monitor or alert users and healthcare providers to cardiac events.
- **Insulin Pumps**: Unauthorized control of an insulin pump could lead to improper dosage administration, either too high or too low, putting the patient at risk of hypoglycemia or hyperglycemia.

In extreme cases, such attacks on life-sustaining devices could be life-threatening, underscoring the urgent need for robust security defenses in these IoT systems.

3.3 Device Functionality Risks and Data Integrity

Apart from data theft, IoT-based health devices can also suffer from "denial of service" attacks, where the device is rendered non-functional. Hackers could overload or disrupt the connection, causing the device to fail at critical times. This raises the issue of **data integrity**—the assurance that the data collected and transmitted by the device is accurate and reliable. Cyberattacks that compromise data integrity can lead to incorrect diagnoses, improper treatments, or missed critical alerts, resulting in potential harm to the patient [11].

3.4 Security Protocols and Defense Mechanisms

To prevent these threats, healthcare providers, manufacturers, and IT professionals must implement stringent security protocols. The main strategies include the following:

1. **Encryption**: Encryption of data in IoT devices ensures its protection during the transfer process. Protocols such as the advanced encryption standard or Rivest–Shamir–Adleman are widely used to prevent cybercriminals from accessing data.
2. **Authentication and Access Control**: When using strong authentication mechanisms, for example biometric verification, two-factor authentication and strong secure passwords, prevent cybercriminals from accessing the devices.

3. **Regular Software Updates**: Cybercriminals often exploit outdated software. Therefore, users and companies need to update the firmware and software of the device regularly in order to address security vulnerabilities.
4. **Intrusion Detection and Prevention**: The deployment of anomaly detection systems using techniques such as fuzzy logic can identify irregular patterns in Device Data, alert to possible violations or tampering.
5. **Device Monitoring and Logging**: Constant monitoring of the device status, connection and data flow can help in the early detection of any unauthorized attempts.

3.5 Importance of Patient Awareness and Education

In addition to technological defenses, educating patients about safe practices with their IoT devices can play a significant role in preventing cyber threats. Patients should be advised on secure internet practices, such as:

- Regularly updating device software and passwords.
- Avoiding public or unsecured Wi-Fi networks.
- Being cautious about sharing data with third-party applications or services.

3.6 Data Privacy and Confidentiality in Wearable Devices

Wearable health devices continuously collect and analyze users' health information. This information is extremely sensitive as it is among the patients' personal data. Information such as users' heart rhythm, blood sugar level or physical activity can be transferred to cloud servers for evaluation by healthcare institutions. However, data privacy and privacy protection pose a major problem in this process [14].

In order to protect the privacy of health data, it is necessary to use strong encryption methods. In addition, it is important to adopt authentication mechanisms and multi-layered security protocols to prevent unauthorized access. Otherwise, cyber attackers can access sensitive information collected through these devices and use this information maliciously.

4 Cybersecurity Protocols Applied for Healthcare IoT Devices

The security of IoT devices used in the healthcare sector is attempted to be ensured with various protocols and standards. These protocols aim to ensure that devices transmit data and perform transactions securely. The main security protocols used to increase the security of IoT-based healthcare devices are as follows:

Encryption Protocols: Encrypting data transmitted from wearable healthcare devices is an important step towards preventing data from being intercepted by third parties [13]. Data Breach Detection Systems: Since IoT-based healthcare devices are constantly connected to the network, security systems that can detect potential data breaches at an early stage are needed. These systems can intervene and prevent the attack if anomalies are detected [15].

4.1 Encryption Protocols

Encryption is a major defense mechanism that transforms data into an impossible-to-read format and provides decryption only with the correct decryption key. In the case of IoT devices in healthcare, proper encryption is the only way to make the data that is subjected to leak and attack and even eavesdropping remain secret. One of the widely adopted symmetric encryption algorithms for data encryption is the advanced encryption standard (AES), which has the advantage of providing a high level of security, a fast operation that makes it suitable for real-time data encryption, and efficiency. So, as an example, let's consider how safety is afforded in AES-256 which is even stronger than brute force attacks. The Rivest-Shamir-Adelman algorithm (RSA) is a public-key encryption method that is most commonly used for secure data transmission. It does so by a pairing of keys: a public key for encryption and private key for decryption, which increases security in situations where distributing Secure Keys is problematic. Lastly, the elliptic curve encryption algorithm (ECC) is a highly effective method of encryption that, even though it is smaller than RSA, guarantees equal amounts of security, thus it is perfectly suited for any mobile device that is constrained by available resources. The ease of processing thus achieved prolongs battery life while keeping the device safe from potential attacks (Table 5).

Table 5. Common Encryption Protocols for Healthcare IoT Devices

Encryption Protocol	Type	Description	Benefits	Use Cases
AES (Advanced Encryption Standard)	Symmetric	Utilizes the same key for encryption and decryption. Highly secure and efficient	High security, fast processing	Real-time data encryption on wearables
RSA (Rivest-Shamir-Adleman)	Asymmetric	Uses a pair of keys (public and private) for secure data transmission	Secure key distribution, robust against attacks	Secure communication between devices and servers
ECC (Elliptic Curve Cryptography)	Asymmetric	Employs smaller key sizes for similar security levels as RSA	Reduced computational load, energy-efficient	Secure data transmission in resource-constrained devices

4.2 Authentication and Authorization

Biometric authentication based on unique biological attributes such as fingerprints, facial recognition, or iris scanning is used to authenticate users, enhancing security and ensuring that access is granted only to the legitimate user. Multi-factor verification also combines two different types of verification, usually something the user knows (password) and something he owns (mobile device or security code). This two-tier approach significantly reduces the risk of unauthorized access. The role-based access management (RBAC) grants access permissions based on the user's role within the organization, ensuring that users can access only the data and functions necessary for their roles, reducing the risk of security breaches [16] (Table 6).

Table 6. Authentication and Authorization Methods for Healthcare IoT Devices

Method	Description	Benefits	Use Cases
Biometric Verification	Uses unique biological traits for user authentication	High security, user convenience	Access control for wearable devices
Two-Factor Authentication (2FA)	Combines two different verification methods for enhanced security	Reduced risk of unauthorized access	Device login, sensitive data access
Role-Based Access Control (RBAC)	Assigns permissions based on user roles within an organization	Minimizes data exposure, scalable management	Healthcare provider access to patient data

4.3 Data Breach Detection Systems

It is of great importance to implement robust systems for detecting data breaches in Internet-based healthcare, given the constant communication between devices connected to the Internet of this type. These systems monitor network traffic and hardware behavior to detect any abnormal changes that may indicate cyber attacks. The threat detection system can be based on two patterns: the first signature-based detection system that detects known threats, and the second exception-based detection system that identifies deviations from normal behavior. The functionality of the threat detection system can be expanded so that it includes not only detection, but also the ability to actively block identified threats. Intrusion prevention system (IPS) provides the ability to block malicious traffic in real time, reducing the impact of cyber attacks. The fuzzy logic is used to deal with uncertainties and inaccuracies in data, which improves the accuracy of exception detection in complex Internet of things environments (Table 7).

4.4 Secure Communication Protocols

Secure protocols for communication are necessary to protect data during its transition between devices of the Internet of things, portals and cloud servers. These protocols ensure that data remains confidential, integrated and reliable during transmission.

Table 7. Data Breach Detection Systems for Healthcare IoT Devices

Detection System	Description	Benefits	Use Cases
Intrusion Detection Systems (IDS)	Monitors network traffic for suspicious activities using signature or anomaly-based methods	Early threat detection, comprehensive monitoring	Network security for healthcare systems
Intrusion Prevention Systems (IPS)	Detects and actively prevents identified threats by blocking malicious traffic	Real-time threat mitigation, enhanced security	Protecting IoT devices from ongoing attacks
Machine Learning-Based Detection	Uses machine learning to analyze data patterns and identify potential breaches	Adaptive to new threats, high accuracy	Continuous monitoring of device behavior
Fuzzy Logic-Based Detection	Utilizes fuzzy logic to manage uncertainties in data, improving anomaly detection	Handles complex and uncertain data, increased accuracy	Detecting nuanced security threats in IoT environments

SSL/TLS protocols create encrypted links between devices and servers, ensuring the security of data sent over the internet from intrusion and manipulation. HTTPS is an extension of the HTTP protocol that uses SSL/TLS to encrypt data exchanged between web browsers and servers (Table 8).

Table 8. Secure Communication Protocols for Healthcare IoT Devices

Protocol	Description	Benefits	Use Cases
SSL/TLS	Establishes encrypted links between devices and servers	Data confidentiality, integrity, and authenticity	Secure data transmission between devices and cloud
HTTPS	Encrypts data exchanged between web browsers and servers	Secure web-based communication	Health applications accessing patient data online
MQTTS	Secures MQTT protocol with SSL/TLS for message transmission	Secure IoT messaging, low latency	Real-time health data streaming to cloud
DTLS	Provides TLS security for datagram-based protocols	Secure real-time communication, low latency	Emergency alert systems, real-time monitoring

4.5 Device Firmware and Software Security

For Internet of Things (IoT) devices to remain safe, regular upgrades and secure firmware are essential. Hackers may use firmware or software flaws to obtain unauthorised access or stop a device from working. Secure Boot, one of the security mechanisms, makes sure that devices boot up with trusted and validated firmware, avoiding the installation of malicious or unauthorised software. Additionally, devices may acquire security fixes and feature enhancements without physical involvement thanks to Over-the-Air (OTA) updates, which enable remote firmware and software upgrades. Additionally, code signing ensures that only authorised updates are installed on devices by using digital signatures to confirm the integrity and validity of updates [18] (Table 9).

Table 9. Firmware and Software Security Measures for Healthcare IoT Devices

Security Measure	Description	Benefits	Use Cases
Secure Boot	Ensures devices boot using only trusted and verified firmware	Prevents unauthorized firmware loading	Initial device startup, firmware integrity
Over-the-Air (OTA) Updates	Enables remote updating of firmware and software to address vulnerabilities	Easy deployment of security patches, minimal downtime	Regular security updates for wearable devices
Code Signing	Verifies the authenticity and integrity of firmware and software updates	Protects against malicious updates	Ensuring legitimate updates are applied to devices

4.6 Network Security Measures

Protecting the network infrastructure that connects IoT devices is essential to prevent unauthorized access and data breaches. Implementing comprehensive network security measures ensures that the entire IoT ecosystem remains secure. The Firewalls Act as a barrier between trusted internal networks and untrusted external networks, controlling incoming and outgoing traffic based on predefined security rules.Virtual Private Networks Create encrypted tunnels for data transmission over public networks, ensuring that data remains secure even when transmitted over unsecured channels. Network Segmentation Divides the network into distinct segments, limiting the spread of potential breaches and containing security incidents within isolated parts of the network (Table 10).

4.7 Comprehensive Security Frameworks

Adopting comprehensive security frameworks ensures that all aspects of IoT device security are addressed systematically. These frameworks provide guidelines and best

Table 10. Network Security Measures for Healthcare IoT Devices

Network Security Measure	Description	Benefits	Use Cases
Firewalls	Controls incoming and outgoing network traffic based on security rules	Blocks unauthorized access, monitors traffic	Protecting internal healthcare networks
Virtual Private Networks (VPNs)	Creates encrypted tunnels for secure data transmission over public networks	Ensures data confidentiality and integrity	Remote access for healthcare professionals
Network Segmentation	Divides the network into separate segments to contain breaches	Limits spread of attacks, enhances security	Isolating critical health data systems from general networks

practices for securing IoT devices throughout their lifecycle [19]. NIST Cybersecurity Framework, Provides a structured approach to man-aging and reducing cybersecurity risks. It consists of five core functions: Identify, Protect, Detect, Respond, and Recover, which guide the implemen-tation of security measures. ISO/IEC 27001 An international standard for information security man-agement systems (ISMS). It outlines require-ments for establishing, imple-menting, maintaining, and continually improving an ISMS, ensuring com-prehensive security coverage (Table 11).

Table 11. Comprehensive Security Frameworks for Healthcare IoT Devices

Framework/Standard	Description	Benefits	Use Cases
NIST Cybersecurity Framework	Provides guidelines for identifying, protecting, detecting, responding, and recovering from cybersecurity threats	Structured risk management, adaptable to various environments	Developing and maintaining IoT security strategies
ISO/IEC 27001	International standard for establishing and maintaining an information security management system (ISMS)	Comprehensive security management, global recognition	Implementing ISMS for healthcare organizations
HIPAA Compliance	U.S. regulation ensuring the protection of patient health information	Legal compliance, enhanced data protection	Managing patient data in healthcare IoT devices

4.8 Implementation Challenges and Best Practices

In addition to continually changing cyber threats, healthcare institutions confront substantial obstacles when implementing cybersecurity policies, including lack of knowledge and budgetary restrictions. Strategic planning and adherence to best practices are necessary to meet these problems. Lack of resources, the difficulty of integrating protocols into internet-connected equipment and healthcare systems, and the ever-evolving threats are some of the main obstacles. Healthcare organisations must implement multi-layered security strategies, provide ongoing training to employees and patients, and keep an eye out for security events on their systems in order to overcome these obstacles. Investment in cutting-edge technology like artificial intelligence for automated response and early threat detection is also crucial, as is cooperation between healthcare providers, device makers, and security specialists.

4.9 Future Directions in IoT Healthcare Security

The rapid progress in the technology of the Internet of things, is leading to an evolution in security measures to be protected. The future of private security in healthcare is focused on how to improve and develop existing protocols, leading to the creation and development of solutions to address new threats. We also know that the eyes are turning towards blockchain to increase security and data protection, which ensures data integrity and therefore makes patient data difficult to manipulate or access. Artificial intelligence and machine learning help detect and address security threats that occur on the system by analyzing data by dividing it into groups to identify patterns that indicate cyber attacks. On the other hand, quantum encryption provides unprecedented high levels of security and protection by taking advantage of the mechanics of quantum encryption, and therefore makes access to data impossible (Table 12).

Table 12. Emerging Technologies in IoT Healthcare Security

Emerging Technology	Description	Benefits	Use Cases
Blockchain	Decentralized ledger technology ensuring data integrity and secure transactions	Tamper-proof records, enhanced data integrity	Secure patient data management, immutable health records
Artificial Intelligence (AI)	Utilizes machine learning algorithms for advanced threat detection and response	Predictive threat detection, automated responses	Real-time monitoring and anomaly detection in IoT devices
Quantum Cryptography	Employs quantum mechanics principles for unbreakable encryption	Unprecedented data security, resistance to quantum attacks	Future-proof encryption for sensitive health data
Zero Trust Architecture	Security model that verifies every access request, regardless of origin	Minimizes risk of unauthorized access, enhanced security posture	Comprehensive access control for healthcare networks

4.10 Anomaly Detection with Fuzzy Logic

The use of anomaly detection in fuzzy logic is considered one of the effective ways to prevent or minimize the harm of cybersecurity threats in healthcare devices using the internet. This is done by first analyzing how the devices work, after which deviations that occur from the expected levels are recorded. Fuzzy logic plays a crucial role by making the system recognize inaccurate data, which in turn makes it easier to accurately detect changes or deviations in the data flow to and from devices. This in turn allows the rapid identification of threats and security breaches that are likely to occur, helping the system to implement preventive measures and enhance the protection and security of the Internet of things in general in the environments of healthcare devices.

5 Conclusion

The artificial intelligence and machine learning-based security solutions can play an important role in detecting anomalies in network environments where IoT devices are constantly connected and in quickly responding to potential attacks. Wearable health devices offer a unique opportunity to continuously monitor the health status of patients and collect data. However, if the security of these devices is neglected, it is inevitable that patient data will be compromised and potentially lead to incorrect treatments. Therefore, healthcare institutions and technology providers should not only develop the technology, but also prioritize the security of this technology. The expansion of the healthcare IoT ecosystem should encourage device manufacturers, software developers, and healthcare providers to cooperate more on security and lead to the adoption of a common security standard in the sector.

It is anticipated that cybersecurity measures will become more widespread and powerful in the healthcare sector in the future. In this context, it is necessary to develop artificial intelligence-based security systems, improve cloud-based data protection solutions, and make security an integrated part of device production processes. In addition, it is of great importance to raise awareness and raise awareness of healthcare professionals and patients on cybersecurity. To prevent data breaches, users should be informed about security measures and encouraged to use their devices securely.

As a result, cybersecurity in the healthcare sector is a complex and multifaceted issue that needs to be addressed at both the individual and institutional levels. While the integration of wearable devices and IoT technologies into healthcare services improves the quality of patient care, cybersecurity vulnerabilities should not be ignored. The healthcare sector must be vigilant against constantly evolving threats and continue to update security protocols in order to protect patient data and security. This process should be seen not only as a technological necessity but also as an ethical responsibility. Ensuring cybersecurity will continue to play a critical role in the sustainability and reliability of healthcare services.

References

1. Alrawais, A., Alhothaily, A., Hu, C., Cheng, X.: Fog computing for the internet of things: security and privacy issues. IEEE Internet Things J. **4**(5), 1125–1134 (2017). https://doi.org/10.1109/JIOT.2017.2684398
2. Badii, B., Neumann, R., Rios, B.: Enhancing security in IoT-based healthcare systems using blockchain technology. J. Med. Syst. **44**(7), 1–12 (2020). https://doi.org/10.1007/s10916-020-01592-3
3. Chen, Y., Yang, K., Wu, Y., Tang, Y.: Privacy-preserving data aggregation for healthcare IoT devices using homomorphic encryption. IEEE Trans. Inf. Forensics Secur. **14**(8), 2132–2145 (2019). https://doi.org/10.1109/TIFS.2019.2912406
4. Ding, C., Bie, R.: Secure data sharing for healthcare IoT using attribute-based encryption and proxy re-encryption. IEEE Access **6**, 25563–25572 (2018). https://doi.org/10.1109/ACCESS.2018.2814528
5. Hossain, M.S., Muhammad, G., Alhamid, M.F.: Security and privacy issues in IoT-based healthcare systems. IEEE Commun. Mag. **55**(1), 50–56 (2017). https://doi.org/10.1109/MCOM.2017.1600641
6. Li, X., Zhang, Y., Wang, J.: A fuzzy logic-based anomaly detection system for healthcare IoT devices. IEEE Sens. J. **21**(5), 6789–6798 (2021). https://doi.org/10.1109/JSEN.2021.3055678
7. Nguyen, T.N., Nguyen, D.H., Vo, T.K.: Machine learning approaches for cybersecurity in IoT-enabled healthcare systems: a survey. IEEE Access **10**, 11234–11254 (2022). https://doi.org/10.1109/ACCESS.2022.3156789
8. Patel, S., Sharma, R.: Blockchain-based secure data sharing framework for healthcare IoT. J. Netw. Comput. Appl. **135**, 1–12 (2019). https://doi.org/10.1016/j.jnca.2019.02.007
9. Rashid, M.H., Khan, S.U.: Enhancing cybersecurity in healthcare IoT using deep learning techniques. IEEE Trans. Industr. Inf. **16**(3), 2004–2013 (2020). https://doi.org/10.1109/TII.2019.2941234
10. Sivathanu, B., Veeraraghavan, M.: Secure and efficient data transmission in healthcare IoT using elliptic curve cryptography. IEEE Trans. Biomed. Eng. **65**(2), 430–440 (2018). https://doi.org/10.1109/TBME.2017.2754321
11. Smith, J., Lee, K.: Privacy-preserving techniques for healthcare data in IoT environments. IEEE J. Biomed. Health Inf. **25**(4), 1456–1465 (2021). https://doi.org/10.1109/JBHI.2021.3078901
12. Tan, W., Liu, Y.: Secure multi-party computation for healthcare IoT data analytics. IEEE Trans. Cloud Comput. **8**(5), 1572–1584 (2020). https://doi.org/10.1109/TCC.2020.2981234
13. Zeng, M., Wang, F., Li, X.: Enhanced asymmetric scalar-product preserving encryption for secure LBS queries in cloud environments. IEEE Trans. Inf. Forensics Secur. **14**(6), 1458–1471 (2019). https://doi.org/10.1109/TIFS.2018.2876543
14. Yang, Z., Liu, J., Zhou, Y.: Verifiable privacy protection scheme for kNN queries in road network environments. IEEE Trans. Depend. Secure Comput. **17**(2), 345–357 (2020). https://doi.org/10.1109/TDSC.2019.2912345
15. Zhu, Y., Li, H., Gao, L.: Efficient privacy-preserving range queries for healthcare IoT using homomorphic encryption. IEEE Internet Things J. **8**(3), 1654–1665 (2021). https://doi.org/10.1109/JIOT.2020.3034567
16. Wan, J., et al.: Wearable IoT enabled real-time health monitoring system. EURASIP J. Wirel. Commun. Network. **2018**(1), 1–10 (2018)
17. HIMSS. Cybersecurity in Healthcare. HIMSS, https://www.himss.org/resources/cybersecurity-healthcare. Accessed 12 Nov 2024

18. AHIMA Journal. Federal Cybersecurity Efforts Seek to Improve Protection of Health Data Journal of AHIMA (2023). https://journal.ahima.org/federal-cybersecurity-efforts-seek-to-improve-protection-of-health-data. Accessed 12 Nov 2024
19. NIST. NIST Cybersecurity Framework 2.0. National Institute of Standards and Technology (2023). https://www.nist.gov/cyberframework. Accessed 12 Nov 2024
20. Smith, J.: Wearable Devices and IoT in Healthcare. Healthcare Technology Today, Tech Publishers (2023)
21. Doe, J.: IoT Integration and Wearable Devices in Healthcare. Healthcare Technology Insights, HealthTech Publishers (2023)

Integrating Artificial Intelligence and Cybersecurity in Healthcare for the Advancements of Industry 5.0

Firoz Khan[1], Lakshmana Kumar Ramasamy[2](✉), Emad Abd Al Rahman[2], and Amala Jayanthi[3]

[1] Center of Information and Computer Science, Ball State University Indiana, Muncie, USA
firoz.khan@bsu.edu
[2] Computer and Information Science, Higher Colleges of Technology, Ras Al Khaimah, United Arab Emirates
{lramasamy,erahman}@hct.ac.ae
[3] Department of Natural Sciences, University of Stirling, Ras Al Khaimah, United Arab Emirates
amala.j@stir.ae

Abstract. In healthcare, AI-driven solutions and digital innovations are reshaping care delivery. AI-powered robots and brain-machine interfaces are playing a significant role, but the challenge lies in improving healthcare without replacing human professionals. The advent of industry 5.0, where humans and machines work together, offers a new perspective. While AI's ability to analyze large amounts of healthcare data is promising, the increased exchange of this information across devices also raises cybersecurity risks. As healthcare evolves with Industry 5.0, the need for strong cybersecurity to protect patient data becomes even more crucial. This paper delves into the integration of AI and cybersecurity into healthcare under Industry 5.0, focusing on their impact and the urgent need for robust security measures.

Keywords: Artificial intelligence · Cyber Security · Cyber threats · Industry 5.0 · Internet of Things · Healthcare

1 Introduction

Technological advancements have greatly improved healthcare systems, enhancing patient outcomes and operational efficiencies. New healthcare products and services emerge rapidly, transforming how care is delivered, managed, and personalized. These changes shape the healthcare sector and push for further investments in medical technologies and innovations. Like in other industries, these technological shifts can be likened to healthcare revolutions, where each wave of innovation brings profound changes. Historically, healthcare has experienced significant transformations due to innovations like medical devices, telemedicine, and electronic health records. Now, the industry stands on the brink of a new era: Industry 4.0, which centers on smart healthcare systems and the digital transformation of medical facilities, introduced in 2011 [1]. Industry 4.0 has sparked extensive discussions in healthcare conferences and research, particularly around smart systems that enhance patient care.

Despite the enthusiasm surrounding Industry 4.0, some experts in the healthcare field argue that it mirrors previous health information technology systems without delivering the transformative impact expected. Critics claim that while much has been discussed, the practical application in healthcare settings has been limited. However, even as Industry 4.0 gains traction, scholars and experts have started conceptualizing Industry 5.0, which is focused on closer integration between technology and healthcare professionals [2]. This new approach has gained support from various governments and researchers globally, setting the stage for a more human-centered healthcare system.

Industry 5.0 represents a shift towards integrating robots and AI with human workers rather than replacing them. AI-based algorithms play a critical role in Industry 5.0, particularly in processing IoT devices' vast, unstructured data [3]. AI, which simulates human intelligence in machines [4], includes applications such as machine learning, speech recognition, and expert systems. As AI's hype grows, many vendors label their products as AI-based, even when they incorporate only one aspect, such as machine learning. AI requires specialized hardware, software, and programming languages like Python, R, and Java.

AI systems work by analyzing large datasets to identify patterns and make predictions. For instance, a chatbot can learn to conduct lifelike conversations by analyzing text chats [5], while an image recognition program can identify and describe objects in photos [6]. AI focuses on three cognitive processes: learning, reasoning, and self-correction. Learning involves gathering data and formulating rules for its transformation into actionable insights. Reasoning applies the best algorithm to achieve a desired result, while self-correction fine-tunes the algorithms to ensure accuracy.

AI's significance lies in its ability to provide businesses with insights and perform tasks faster and with fewer errors than humans, particularly in repetitive, detail-oriented activities. For instance, AI can analyze large volumes of legal documents to ensure accuracy. This has led to efficiency gains and opened new business opportunities for larger companies. For example, Uber has become one of the world's largest companies by using machine learning to predict when and where people will need rides, allowing drivers to be in position ahead of time [7].

In Industry 5.0, cybersecurity becomes increasingly crucial due to the interconnectedness of devices and systems, which makes them vulnerable to malicious attacks. As data is transferred between devices like cobots, cyber threats pose a significant risk [8]. Securing critical systems and sensitive data from cyberattacks is vital for the success of Industry 5.0. The increasing sophistication of cyber threats has made cybersecurity a critical issue, as demonstrated by the average cost of a data breach reaching $8.64 million in the United States in 2020 [9]. Cybercriminals often target personally identifiable information (PII), such as names, addresses, and Social Security numbers, to sell on the dark web. The exposure of such information can damage a company's reputation, lead to regulatory fines, and result in legal action.

To combat these risks, businesses are adopting comprehensive cybersecurity strategies that incorporate advanced analytics, AI, and machine learning to detect and respond to threats in real time. Industry 5.0, by integrating AI with cybersecurity, offers significant advantages over Industry 4.0. These advanced technologies can identify vulnerabilities, mitigate risks, and enhance operational security, ensuring the smooth progression of digital industrial transformation.

There have been several surveys on Industry 5.0 that provide valuable insights into its development. Maddikunta et al. [10] offered the first-ever discussion on Industry 5.0, exploring its applications in intelligent healthcare, cloud manufacturing, supply chain management, and production. The authors also reviewed supporting technologies such as edge computing, digital twins, collaborative robots, blockchain, and 6G networks. Zeb et al. [11] examined whether computational intelligence and next-generation wireless networks could meet Industry 5.0's communication and processing demands. They reviewed emerging technologies like open radio access networks and software service architectures, identifying challenges and research gaps. Patil et al. [12] focused on the human-machine collaboration in Industry 5.0, emphasizing that prioritizing the human touch in this revolution would make work more efficient and adaptable.

This paper contributes to the ongoing discussion by (1) introducing Industry 5.0 and its relevance to healthcare, (2) summarizing the role of AI in Industry 5.0 healthcare applications, and (3) providing an overview of cybersecurity's growing importance in the healthcare industry during this new industrial era.

The paper is structured as follows: Sect. 2 introduces Industry 5.0, Sect. 3 discusses AI in Industry 5.0 with a focus on healthcare, Sect. 4 covers cybersecurity in healthcare, Section 5 explores open research challenges, and concludes the paper. Overview of Industry 5.0.

1.1 Industrial Revolutions

The First Industrial Revolution began in the 1780s with the adoption of mechanical energy from water, steam, coal, and gas [13]. The Second Industrial Revolution in the 1870s introduced mass production and assembly lines driven by electricity [14]. The Third Industrial Revolution, in the 1970s, saw the rise of automation in manufacturing through electronics and information technologies (IT) [15]. In the Fourth Industrial Revolution, IoT and cloud computing connected the physical and virtual worlds via cyber-physical systems (CPS) [16]. Though Industry 4.0 is still evolving, leaders foresee Industry 5.0, where human intelligence re-integrates with manufacturing [17]. By 2030, an estimated 7.5 billion people are expected to have Internet access, spurring further technological advancements [18].

1.2 Market Dynamics and Technological Integration

Manufacturing must adapt to rapidly shifting market demands, necessitating production lines that are flexible, smart, and scalable. Integration between providers, assembly lines, and consumers is increasingly essential, achieved primarily through IoT—the backbone of Industry 4.0 [19]. The Fourth Industrial Revolution builds on CPS and IoT to enable real-time communication between systems, generating large data sets that require secure cloud storage solutions. Industry 4.0 has significantly reduced production and logistics costs while improving quality management [20].

Key drivers of Industry 4.0 include:

- Widespread IoT connectivity
- Digital twins for real-world applications
- Efficient production lines and smart goods
- Connectivity between business and manufacturing sectors

The implementation of CPS, IoT, and big data has reduced production costs by 1030%, logistics costs by 10–30%, and quality management expenditures by 10–20% [21].

1.3 What is Industry 5.0 and Why is it Necessary?

Industry 4.0's primary focus on automation and operational efficiency overlooks the human cost associated with technological advancement. This issue will become more apparent as Industry 4.0 continues to evolve, potentially sparking pushback from labor groups and policymakers. This opposition will make Industry 5.0 necessary. The environmental impact of industrial processes is another area that Industry 5.0 seeks to address, with companies increasingly focused on reducing waste and negative ecological consequences. Despite progress in AI-driven environmental sustainability efforts, Industry 4.0 does not strongly prioritize environmental protection. Industry 5.0 is expected to fill this gap, driving sustainability efforts [22].

Industry 5.0 will bring human workers back to factory floors, where they will collaborate with robots, combining human creativity and machine intelligence to enhance efficiency. The focus of Industry 5.0 shifts from automation to collaboration between humans and autonomous robots. Cobots—collaborative robots—will assist human workers in a way that improves safety, reduces fear, and fosters a sense of partnership [23]. Cobots will be designed to understand and predict human actions, assisting with tasks as needed and operating safely in human environments.

Cobots will learn from human operators by observing their work and predicting their intentions. For example, a cobot might anticipate a worker's need for a specific component and retrieve it in advance, streamlining the workflow [24]. Cobots will transform manufacturing by enabling humans to work alongside robots that comprehend and act on human intent. Industry 5.0 will likely create new roles, such as Chief Robotics Officer (CRO), responsible for optimizing human-robot collaboration and ensuring safety [25].

1.4 Technologies Driving Industry 5.0

Networked Sensor Data Industry 5.0 will rely heavily on networked sensors for real-time data collection and analysis. These sensors will enable faster assessments and customization in manufacturing while reducing network latency and overload. By processing data locally, networked sensors will provide distributed intelligence across the system, enhancing manufacturing efficiency [26].

Simulation and Digital Twins Digital twins—virtual models of systems, products, or services—bridge the gap between the physical and virtual worlds. They allow manufacturers to simulate production processes, monitor performance, and predict potential issues before they occur. Digital twins offer significant benefits by reducing downtime, minimizing waste, and optimizing system design [27].

Shopfloor Trackers Real-time monitoring through shopfloor trackers links production orders to sales, enabling more effective resource management and operational improvement. These trackers can help reduce waste and prevent theft, optimizing the manufacturing process [28].

Virtual Training Virtual training offers a safe and cost-effective way to develop new skills in simulated environments. This method is particularly useful in hazardous industries where real-world training could pose risks. The use of haptic technologies, such as the Universal Motion Simulator (UMS), enhances virtual training by providing realistic touch feedback, allowing trainees to experience lifelike conditions without physical danger [29, 30].

Intelligent Autonomous Systems Autonomous systems in Industry 5.0 will depend on advanced AI to perform tasks independently, enhancing manufacturing efficiency. AI algorithms like deep learning will enable robots to make decisions and adapt to changing conditions, ensuring that processes run smoothly with minimal human intervention. Autonomous systems will become increasingly intelligent as they learn from data and improve their decision-making capabilities [32].

Advances in Sensing and Cognition Cobots will require sophisticated sensing and cognitive abilities to effectively collaborate with humans. Advances in machine vision, deep learning, and reinforcement learning will enable cobots to predict human intentions and take proactive actions to assist in tasks. Cobots will be able to understand their environment and make decisions that improve safety and efficiency on the factory floor [33].

Human Brain-Computer Interaction Technologies like functional near-infrared spectroscopy (fNIRS) offer new possibilities for human-robot interaction by allowing machines to interpret human brain signals. For example, a cobot equipped with a braincomputer interface could assist a surgeon by responding to brain signals in real-time, enhancing precision and reducing the cognitive load on the human operator [31]. Such advancements in brain-computer interaction will make cobots even more effective collaborators in a variety of industries, from healthcare to manufacturing.

2 Artificial Intelligence in Industry 5.0

Industry 5.0 represents a major advancement from Industry 4.0, focusing on combining human creativity with advanced, intelligent machines to enhance production and operational efficiency. Unlike Industry 4.0, which emphasized automation and data exchange, Industry 5.0 integrates smart technologies and human insight to improve productivity.

2.1 AI's Role in Industry 5.0

AI is crucial in Industry 5.0 for several reasons. First, it significantly enhances data analysis capabilities. AI models can process and analyze vast amounts of unstructured data generated by Internet of Things (IoT) devices, leading to better decision-making and operational improvements. Second, AI facilitates effective collaboration between humans and robots. By leveraging technologies such as IoT and big data, robots can perform tasks with minimal human intervention, thereby increasing efficiency and effectiveness. Third, AI improves smart environments. Intelligent sensors embedded in devices in smart cities and homes gather data that AI analyzes to optimize services and resource management.

2.2 AI Techniques in Industry 5.0

Machine Learning (ML) for Intelligent Sensing: ML models are used to identify patterns and make predictions from data collected by intelligent sensors. Active learning techniques, for example, dynamically enhance the range of classifications a model can recognize, adapting to new data in real time.

Decision Trees (DT): Decision trees are employed to classify data by evaluating various attributes to determine the best way to split the data. This method is useful in applications such as pattern recognition and healthcare management.

Random Forests (RF): RF models consist of multiple decision trees that vote on classifications. By averaging the outcomes of these trees, RF enhances classification accuracy and is effective in detecting unauthorized devices in IoT environments.

Clustering Algorithms:

- K-means: This algorithm clusters data into groups based on similarities. It is known for its speed and scalability, making it suitable for large datasets.
- DBSCAN: This algorithm clusters data based on density, which helps in identifying anomalies and patterns in noisy datasets.

One-Class Support Vector Machine (OC-SVM): OC-SVM detects outliers by creating boundaries around normal data. It is useful in identifying anomalies in network traffic and sensor data.

Ensemble Learning (EL): EL combines multiple learning models to improve accuracy and stability. It is employed in tasks such as intrusion detection and real-time decision making in IoT environments.

Neural Networks (NN): Neural networks, particularly feed-forward neural networks (FFNN), are used for complex tasks such as feature extraction and decision-making in IoT applications. They are capable of handling large datasets and making predictions efficiently.

Support Vector Machines (SVM): SVMs classify data by finding the optimal hyperplane that separates different classes. They are effective in analyzing large datasets and detecting intrusions.

Internet of Intelligent Things (IoIT): IoIT extends IoT by integrating intelligent sensors and networks, creating interactive and intelligent systems. Applying social networking techniques to IoT enhances connectivity and collaboration among devices and users.

Principal Component Analysis (PCA): PCA reduces data dimensionality while retaining variance, aiding in data visualization and preprocessing in machine learning.

Bagging: Bagging improves the accuracy and stability of machine learning models by training on multiple subsets of data and averaging the results. This technique is applicable to various models, including decision trees and neural networks.

Artificial Intelligence in Analytics: AI enhances data processing capabilities, leading to improved decision-making. Analytics 4.0 involves using AI models and machine learning techniques to advance data analysis.

Deep Learning for Analytics: Deep learning techniques are increasingly used in IoT applications to process large volumes of data and make real-time predictions. These methods are crucial for applications in healthcare, smart cities, and other areas.

Edge Computing: Edge computing processes data locally on IoT devices instead of sending it all to the cloud, reducing latency and bandwidth use. It addresses the challenges of handling real-time data streams and supports applications that require immediate data processing.

Federated Learning: Federated learning trains machine learning models across decentralized devices without transferring raw data to a central server. This approach improves data privacy and enables models to learn from local data while maintaining a global model.

3 Cyber Security in Industry 5.0

In Industry 5.0, where devices like collaborative robots (cobots) exchange data, ensuring cyber security is crucial due to the increased risk of malicious attacks. As industries adopt more connected and intelligent technologies, addressing cyber security issues becomes imperative to safeguard digital transformation.

3.1 Characterizing and Measuring Maliciousness

Understanding malicious intent is essential for mitigating cyber threats. Historically, cybersecurity experts have explored how human malice impacts cyber environments, assessing insider threats based on skill and financial motives. Human malice can manifest at micro, meso, and macro levels, each posing potential risks to cyber security. Research into these levels is limited, but they are critical in determining how individuals' personalities and behaviors influence cyber threats. Malicious behavior is often a socio-technical issue, making it important to integrate human factors into cyber security assessments. Challenges include developing standardized methods for evaluating maliciousness and using ontologies to uncover elements leading to cyber-related threats.

3.2 Risk Scenarios

Cyber-attacks in industrial contexts can range from malicious applications halting production processes to social engineering tactics exploiting human traits to bypass security measures. Attacks might involve implanting harmful data packets into systems, disrupting production lines, or stealing sensitive information. Traditional security concerns are now complemented by new risks associated with connected production, which can lead to financial losses, product quality degradation, and worker safety issues. In Industry

5.0, the focus has shifted from mere data confidentiality to protecting the integrity and functionality of physical processes. IoT devices, which are often vulnerable, can lead to severe outcomes like facility damage or even fatalities. Ensuring the security of these devices is crucial to prevent significant financial and operational impacts.

3.3 AI-Based Trustworthiness in IoT

The Internet of Things (IoT) has expanded rapidly, bringing new challenges related to data security and privacy. While IoT can enhance human life, it also introduces vulnerabilities such as viruses and unwanted content. Securing IoT systems involves protecting data across networks and ensuring privacy through robust security measures, including cryptographic algorithms, firewalls, and intrusion prevention systems.

Emerging technologies like machine learning, deep learning, and blockchain can enhance IoT security. However, issues like unauthorized data collection and sales by device providers highlight the need for stringent data ethics and security practices.

3.4 Cybersecurity Concerns in Industry 5.0, Especially Collaborative Robots

Collaborative robots (cobots), designed to work alongside humans, face unique cybersecurity challenges. Despite efforts to ensure their safety, vulnerabilities in cobots can endanger human workers. Common security threats include:

- Altered Output: Hackers can modify robot programming to produce defective parts, impacting product integrity.
- Ransomware: Attackers may seize control of cobots, demanding payment to restore functionality.
- Physical Damage: Compromised robots can cause physical harm to people or equipment.
- Production Disruption: Hacked cobots can cause bottlenecks and damage products.
- Data Theft: Hackers may exploit cobot controllers to steal sensitive information.

The impact of such breaches can be severe, affecting safety, product integrity, and accuracy. Subtle changes in a robot's programming or calibration can go unnoticed but have dangerous consequences. For example, hackers might alter calibration parameters, disrupt production logic, or mislead users about the robot's status, potentially leading to severe injuries.

3.5 Do's and Don'ts to Protect Your Cobots' Cybersecurity

To safeguard cobots in Industry 5.0, companies should adopt specific practices: Prioritize Cyber Security from the Start: Address cyber security early in the planning stages and adjust strategies as needed.

- Avoid Blanket Techniques: Tailor security measures for cobots rather than applying the same methods used for traditional industrial robots.
- Consider Various Scenarios: Use scenario planning to identify potential vulnerabilities and improve cyber security strategies.

- Protect Company Data: Implement comprehensive security measures to safeguard data from IoT devices and prevent unauthorized access or breaches.
- Choose Secure Vendors: Select cobot manufacturers with robust security protocols and ongoing updates for emerging vulnerabilities.
- Incorporate Employee Feedback: Train employees to recognize and report unusual cobot behavior, as they may detect issues others might miss.

Cyber security awareness and proactive measures are essential to mitigate risks associated with cobots and other Industry 5.0 technologies. Ensuring robust security practices helps prevent significant harm and maintains the safe and efficient operation of industrial systems.

4 Opportunities and Challenges of Industry 5.0

4.1 Opportunities

- Job Creation and Efficiency: The integration of next-generation technologies in Industry 5.0 is expected to enhance healthcare employment by automating routine tasks while creating new opportunities for skilled professionals, such as AI specialists, data analysts, and cybersecurity experts. This transition will allow healthcare workers to focus on more critical tasks, improving overall efficiency in patient care and medical operations.
- Customization and Personalization: Enhanced automation enables more personalized healthcare, offering patients tailored treatment plans, medications, and services. This can improve patient outcomes and satisfaction by addressing individual needs more precisely, fostering loyalty to healthcare providers and institutions.
- Improved Safety and Innovation: Collaborative robots (COBOTs) can handle hazardous tasks, such as assisting in surgeries or managing biohazard materials, thus enhancing the safety of healthcare workers. Industry 5.0 also provides opportunities for startups and innovative companies to develop new medical devices, diagnostic tools, and treatment methods, driving forward healthcare innovations.
- Human-Machine Interaction: Industry 5.0 advances research in human-machine collaboration, offering healthcare providers new ways to interact with technology, such as AI-powered diagnostic tools and robotic assistants. It also supports the expansion of telemedicine and remote care, improving access to specialized healthcare services, particularly in underserved or remote areas.

4.2 Challenges

- Workforce Disparities: Automation in Industry 5.0 healthcare systems risks widening the gap between high-skilled healthcare professionals, such as AI specialists and data scientists, and lower-skilled healthcare workers. Addressing this disparity through upskilling and education is essential to ensure equitable workforce development.
- Skill Development: The advanced technologies in Industry 5.0 require healthcare workers to undergo substantial training to effectively integrate and utilize AI, robotics, and data analytics systems. Both existing healthcare professionals and new entrants must adapt to these sophisticated tools to maintain efficient care delivery.

- Cybersecurity Risks: With increased connectivity and data sharing in healthcare through IoT devices and AI-driven systems, the risk of cyber threats becomes more severe. Ensuring robust cybersecurity measures is crucial to protect sensitive patient data and maintain trust in digital healthcare systems.
- Investment and Infrastructure: Fully realizing the potential of Industry 5.0 in healthcare requires significant investment in new technology, medical devices, and supporting infrastructure. This poses challenges, especially for smaller healthcare providers and startups that may struggle with the cost of implementation.
- Data Management and Integration: Managing large amounts of high-quality healthcare data from various sources, such as wearable devices, electronic health records, and diagnostic tools, remains complex. Ensuring smooth integration and maintaining data integrity across healthcare systems is vital for patient outcomes.
- Regulatory and Strategic Adaptation: The high degree of automation and AI in healthcare challenges existing regulatory frameworks, necessitating new guidelines for accountability, patient safety, and data privacy. Healthcare organizations must also adapt their business models to meet evolving patient needs and preferences in this increasingly digital landscape.

5 Conclusion

Industry 5.0 in healthcare emphasizes the collaboration between humans and machines to enhance patient care, operational efficiency, and personalized treatment. By integrating big data, AI, IoT, cloud computing, and collaborative robots (COBOTS), Industry 5.0 aims to improve the quality of healthcare services and streamline medical processes while offering more personalized and efficient care options for patients. However, it also presents challenges, such as the need for advanced skill development for healthcare professionals and heightened cybersecurity risks due to increased connectivity and data sharing. Despite these challenges, Industry 5.0 is expected to transform healthcare through closer human-robot collaboration, improving patient outcomes and operational efficiency. Integrating AI and cybersecurity will play a critical role in advancing smart, secure, and patient-centered healthcare systems for the future.

References

1. Oztemel, E., Gursev, S.: Literature review of Industry 4.0 and related technologies. J. Intell. Manuf. **31**(1), 127–182 (2020)
2. Xu, X., Lu, Y., Vogel-Heuser, B., Wang, L.: Industry 4.0 and Industry 5.0—inception, conception and perception. J. Manuf. Syst. **61**, 530–535 (2021)
3. Chander, B., Pal, S., De, D., Buyya, R.: Artificial intelligence-based Internet of things for industry 5.0. In: Pal, S., De, D., Buyya, R. (eds.) Artificial Intelligence-based Internet of Things Systems, pp. 3–45. Springer, Cham (2022). https://doi.org/10.1007/978-3-030-87059-1_1
4. Lele, A.: Artificial intelligence (AI). In: Lele, A. (ed.) Disruptive technologies for the militaries and security, pp. 139–154. Springer, Singapore (2019). https://doi.org/10.1007/978-981-13-3384-2_8

5. Haristiani, N.: Artificial Intelligence (AI) chatbot as language learning medium: an inquiry. In: Journal of Physics: Conference Series, vol. 1387, no. 1, p. 012020. IOP Publishing (2019)
6. Robertson, S., Azizpour, H., Smith, K., Hartman, J.: Digital image analysis in breast pathology—from image processing techniques to artificial intelligence. Transl. Res. **194**, 19–35 (2018)
7. Bresnahan, T., Yin, P.L.: Adoption of new information and communications technologies in the workplace today. Innov. Policy Econ. **17**(1), 95–124 (2017)
8. Sarker, I.H., Kayes, A.S.M., Badsha, S., Alqahtani, H., Watters, P., Ng, A.: Cybersecurity data science: an overview from machine learning perspective. J. Big data **7**(1), 1–29 (2020)
9. Statista. 2022. Data breach: average US organizational cost 2020 | Statista. https://www.statista.com/statistics/273575/average-organizational-cost-incurred-by-a-data-breach/. Accessed 17 June 2022
10. Maddikunta, P.K.R., et al.: Industry 5.0: a survey on enabling technologies and potential applications. J. Ind. Inf. Integrat. **26**, 100257 (2022)
11. Zeb, S., e al.: Industry 5.0 is coming: a survey on intelligent nextg wireless networks as technological enablers. arXiv preprint arXiv:2205.09084 (2022)
12. Patil, A.R., Thakur, K., Gandhi, K., Savale, V., Sayyed, N.: A review on Industry 5.0: the techno-social revolution. Int. J. Mech. Eng. **7**(5), 1–5 (2022)
13. Mohajan, H.: The first industrial revolution: creation of a new global human era (2019)
14. Kumar, A., Kumar, S.: Industry 4.0: evolution, opportunities and challenges. Int. J. Res. Bus. Stud. **5**(1), 139–148 (2020)
15. Afolalu, S.A., Ikumapayi, O.M., Abdulkareem, A., Soetan, S.B., Emetere, M.E., Ongbali, S.O.: Enviable roles of manufacturing processes in sustainable fourth industrial revolution–a case study of mechatronics. Mater. Today: Proc. **44**, 2895–2901 (2021)
16. Haleem, A., Javaid, M., Singh, R.P., Suman, R., Rab, S.: Holography and its applications for industry 4.0: an overview. In: Internet of Things and Cyber-Physical Systems (2022)
17. Noble, S.M., Mende, M., Grewal, D., Parasuraman, A.: The fifth industrial revolution: how harmonious human–machine collaboration is triggering a retail and service [r]evolution. J. Retail. **98**, 199–208 (2022)
18. Freeze, D.: Humans on the Internet will triple from 2015 to 2022 and hit 6 Billion. Cybercrime Magazine (2019). Accessed 17 June 2022. https://cybersecurityventures.com/how-many-internet-users-will-the-world-have-in-2022-and-in-2030/
19. Xu, M., David, J.M., Kim, S.H.: The fourth industrial revolution: opportunities and challenges. Int. J. Finan. Res. **9**(2), 90–95 (2018)
20. Pivoto, D.G., de Almeida, L.F., da Rosa Righi, R., Rodrigues, J.J., Lugli, A.B., Alberti, A.M.: Cyber-physical systems architectures for industrial internet of things applications in Industry 4.0: a literature review. J. Manuf. Syst. **58**, 176–192 (2021)
21. Ortiz, J.H., Marroquin, W.G., Cifuentes, L.Z.: Industry 4.0: current status and future trends. Intechopen.com (2019). Accessed 17 June 2022. https://www.intechopen.com/chapters/70465
22. Nahavandi, S.: Industry 5.0—a human-centric solution. Sustainability **11**(16), 4371 (2019)
23. Mourtzis, D., Angelopoulos, J., Panopoulos, N.: Operator 5.0: a survey on enabling technologies and a framework for digital manufacturing based on extended reality. J. Mach. Eng. **22** (2022)
24. Pinti, P., et al.: A review on the use of wearable functional near-infrared spectroscopy in naturalistic environments. Jpn. Psychol. Res. **60**(4), 347–373 (2018)
25. Bigan, C.: Trends in teaching artificial intelligence for industry 5.0. In: Draghici, A., Ivascu, L. (eds.) Sustainability and Innovation in Manufacturing Enterprises: Indicators, Models and Assessment for Industry 5.0, pp. 257–274. Springer, Singapore (2022). https://doi.org/10.1007/978-981-16-7365-8_10

26. Rababah, B., Eskicioglu, R.: Distributed intelligence model for IoT applications based on neural networks. Int. J. Comput. Netw. Inf. Secur. **13**(3), 1–14 (2021)
27. Aheleroff, S., Xu, X., Zhong, R.Y., Lu, Y.: Digital twin as a service (DTaaS) in industry 4.0: an architecture reference model. Adv. Eng. Inf. **47**, 101225 (2021)
28. Rácz-Szabó, A., Ruppert, T., Bántay, L., Löcklin, A., Jakab, L., Abonyi, J.: Real-time locating system in production management. Sensors **20**(23), 6766 (2020)
29. Rizzo, A., Thomas Koenig, S., Talbot, T.B.: Clinical results using virtual reality. J. Technol. Hum. Serv. **37**(1), 51–74 (2019)
30. Patent Owner, Universal Motion Simulator. US Patent Patent US20160096276A1; Application 14/872,177 (2016). https://patents.google.com/patent/US20160096276A1/en. Accessed 17 June 2022
31. Fahim, S., et al.: Augmented reality and virtual reality in dentistry: highlights from the current research. Appl. Sci. **12**(8), 3719 (2022)
32. Sarker, I.H.: Deep learning: a comprehensive overview on techniques, taxonomy, applications and research directions. SN Comput. Sci. **2**(6), 1–20 (2021)
33. Sahoo, D., Pham, Q., Lu, J., Hoi, S.C.: Online deep learning: Learning deep neural networks on the fly. arXiv preprint arXiv:1711.03705 (2017)

Author Index

A
Aksoy, Bekir 47
Al Rahman, Emad Abd 198
Andreozzi, Viviana 34
Arturo, Domínguez-Miranda Sergio 87

B
Binu, Akhil 108

C
Catalano, Claudio 34
Cosoli, Gloria 117

D
Dass, Rahul 22

E
Eylence, Muzaffer 47

F
Faisal, Mohammed Ridha Faisa 182

G
Gawali, Shubhangi 108
Goveas, Neena 108

H
Handur-Kulkarni, Aditya 108

J
Jain, Ishna 22
Jayanthi, Amala 198

K
Khan, Firoz 198
Kumar, Shrawan 3

L
Liguori, Sara 34
Lin, Shufan 132

M
Maresca, Luca 34
Milojevic, Dusko 159

N
Nisevic, Maja 159

O
Özmen, Mustafa Melikşah 47

P
Panni, Luna 117
Pontillo, Gabriele 34
Putta, Mamatha 59

R
Rachuri, Harish Kumar 22
Rajaram, Bharghava 22
Ramasamy, Lakshmana Kumar 198
Rana, Shashank 108
Roman, Rodriguez-Aguilar 87

S
Sandbulte, Jomara 59
Scalise, Lorenzo 117

T
Thakur, Bharti 3
Tsai, Zsehong 132

The manufacturer's authorised representative in the EU is Springer Nature Customer Service Centre GmbH, Europaplatz 3, 69115 Heidelberg, Germany. If you have any concerns regarding our products, please contact ProductSafety@springernature.com

Printed and bound by CPI Group (UK) Ltd, Croydon, CR0 4YY
26/03/2026
02078976-0002